ARE YOU LOOKING FOR *NATURAL* RELIEF?

- Do you suffer from the pain of arthritis?
- Do you put up with chronic back or neck pain?
- Are you bothered by allergies?
- Do you have skin problems?
- Do you experience frequent heartburn?
- Would you like to feel better than you do now?

YOU MAY NOT BE GETTING ENOUGH OF MSM, THE NATURAL, WATER-SOLUBLE NUTRIENT THE BODY REQUIRES.

MSM

THE NATURAL PAIN RELIEF REMEDY

DEBORAH MITCHELL
Foreword by Steven J. Bock, M.D.

A Lynn Sonberg Book

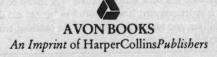

AVON BOOKS
An Imprint of HarperCollins*Publishers*

The ideas, procedures, and suggestions in this book are intended to supplement, not replace, the medical advice of a trained medical professional. All matters regarding your health require medical supervision. Consult your physician before adopting the suggestions in this book, as well as about any condition that may require diagnosis or medical attention. The author and publisher disclaim any liability arising directly or indirectly from the use of this book.

This book is intended to provide selected information about MSM (methylsulfonylmethane), a dietary sulfur supplement. Research about MSM is ongoing and subject to conflicting interpretations. As a result, there is no guarantee that what we know about this subject won't change with time.

AVON BOOKS
An Imprint of HarperCollins*Publishers*
10 East 53rd Street
New York, New York 10022-5299

Copyright © 1999 by Lynn Sonberg Book Associates
Published by arrangement with Lynn Sonberg Book Associates
Library of Congress Catalog Card Number: 99-94801
ISBN: 0-380-80899-4
www.avonbooks.com

First Avon Books printing: December 2000
First Wholecare printing: September 1999

Avon Trademark Reg. U.S. Pat. Off. and in Other Countries, Marca Registrada, Hecho en U.S.A.
HarperCollins® is a trademark of HarperCollins Publishers Inc.

Printed in the U.S.A.

10 9 8 7 6 5 4 3

❀

Contents

※

Foreword

The human body and all its intricate functions never cease to amaze us. Few days go by without the news media reporting on new findings concerning what we should and shouldn't eat, which vitamins to take or not take, how much sleep we should or should not get, and on and on.

Doubtless you've heard or read about a new dietary supplement called MSM. Natural dietary sulfur, or MSM, is not something new; indeed, it's been the subject of many animal studies and clinical trials since the 1950s. That's also about the time a substance called DMSO was in the news. You may remember or may have read about how DMSO was taken by thousands of people to relieve various types of pain. Although

DMSO was effective, the Food and Drug Administration (FDA) eventually approved its use in humans for only one medical condition, and it faded from the public eye.

In the meantime, MSM, a derivative of DMSO, was under scrutiny. Indications were that MSM not only offered the benefits of DMSO, it also did not possess its biggest downfall: a strong, persistent fishlike odor. Now, years later, stories from patients and doctors alike are pouring in: MSM relieves the pain and inflammation of arthritis, safely and odor-free. These reports may prove to be welcome news to the more than 40 million Americans who suffer with this disease. People with gastrointestinal problems, muscle cramps, allergies and asthma.

A certain amount of skepticism often follows the report of any new scientific discovery or study finding, especially one that has the potential to affect the daily lives of millions of people. This can be a healthy response, because it may stimulate discussion and prompt those who were responsible for the discovery to defend their work. Often the products of such discussions are further proof of the value of the work, expanded opportunities to use it, and perhaps ways to improve it. This is proving to be the case with MSM: as more people hear about it, discuss it, and use it, their enthusiasm is fueling more research, more interest from physicians, and the production of more information about it.

That leads you to the book you now have in your hand, *MSM: The Natural Pain Relief Remedy*, a concise, comprehensive, yet readable book that poses and answers the questions you and many others have about MSM: what it is, where it came from, why there is such sudden interest in this little-known mineral, what it's good for, as well as what other natural treatments may be used with it.

The recent attention given to MSM and the public's demand for the product is just one illustration of the burgeoning interest in safe, natural remedies and the dissatisfaction with drugs that either don't provide relief or are associated with bothersome or debilitating side effects. MSM offers people the opportunity to be good to themselves: to remedy a nutritional deficiency, relieve pain, reduce inflammation, or help restore nutritional balance.

As a traditionally trained physician who has integrated conventional medicine and alternative medicine for more than fifteen years, I have treated or consulted with thousands of people who have arthritis. In many cases, I prescribe or recommend MSM, and the response has been excellent. Some patients take MSM along with prescription medications and eventually reduce the amount of drugs they need for pain relief; others can vitually eliminate their reliance on conventional medications. Along with MSM I find that daily doses of a ginger extract provides much needed relief for these patients.

Given the nutritionally deprived state of much of our food supply and the poor dietary habits of many Americans, it is nearly impossible to remedy mineral deficiencies with food. Dietary sulfur, or MSM, is especially difficult to obtain from the diet because it is lost when food is processed. A sulfur or MSM deficiency is likely much more widespread than imagined. Supplements have become necessary.

MSM: The Natural Pain Relief Remedy is an important book because it presents an overview of the MSM story—including what this important supplement can and cannot do—so readers can make up their own minds about whether they want to take it. MSM is an optional treatment for the millions of people who suffer daily with the pain and frustration of arthritis, a treatment they can use alone or along with their current therapy. To further help people make informed choices, this book offers the latest information on other natural remedies to treat arthritis, including glucosamine, chondroitan, ginger extracts, and various nutritional supplements; and current conventional drugs, which include nonsteroidal anti-inflammatory drugs and the new super aspirins. This book helps individuals place control of their health in their own hands.

This book does not portray MSM as a miracle cure. It recognizes that MSM will help many people but not everyone. The only true miracle is the one that goes on every day in the human body—the incredibly complex interrelationships between cells, between mind and body—that make life possible. MSM is *an* answer, and indications are that it is a much-awaited one for many people, especially those with arthritis.

MSM: The Natural Pain Relief Remedy lets people know they have many options when it comes to their health. It answers a great many questions about MSM and natural products you can take to complement it, and provides a balanced perspective of the pros and cons of this exciting and important addition to the supplement market.

Steven J. Bock, M.D.

❀

ONE

❀

Why All the Fuss Over MSM?

Perhaps you've heard about MSM from a magazine article, or seen it featured on a television show. Or maybe you've heard about MSM through a friend or coworker who's had experience with it—someone whose arthritis vanished, or who was able to stop taking aspirin or Tylenol after years of steady pill-popping. Perhaps you've even heard about other conditions that responded to this mysterious new substance: diabetes, skin problems, even chronic infections. You're intrigued by the idea of using a nutritional substance, instead of a drug, to foster your health. You'd rather build a healthy body from the inside out than mask the pain and symptoms of bodily malfunctioning with pharmaceuticals. You've probably heard that up to 80 percent of the costs of managed health care in America can be traced to chronic conditions—and you know there must be a better way.

So you've picked up this book looking for answers about MSM. What is it, exactly? What do we know about how it works in the body? Can we believe the stories we've heard about such far-reaching health benefits? And can we really be sure that it's both safe and effective?

What is MSM?

MSM is the short name for methylsulfonylmethane, a complicated-sounding chemical that's really a fairly simple thing. It's a water-soluble compound that's found in all living things on Earth: plants, animals, fish, even algae. MSM is an organic form of sulfur, the element most of us last heard about in high school chemistry class. Like the mineral sulfur, MSM is a nutrient—a specific type of dietary sulfur that our bodies require in our diet to perform their essential functions. It's not a drug. Instead, it functions as part of a complex symphony of vitamins, minerals, and other compounds that work together to facilitate virtually every bodily process you can imagine, from circulation to digestion, infection-fighting to wound healing.

Is MSM like sulfa or sulfites?

Because MSM is a form of sulfur, you might mistake it for one of several other compounds with similar names, yet very different characteristics. For example, when you think of sulfur, you might also think of sulfa, or more specifically, sulfa drugs, which are also known as sulfonamides. Sulfa drugs, such as erythromycin and sulfacytine, are powerful antibacterial pharmaceuticals used to treat systemic infections. Sulfites, which are a class of food preservatives with no nutritive value, are found under various names, such as sodium sulfite, sodium bisulfite, and potassium bisulfite. Neither sulfa drugs nor sulfites has much to do with MSM.

Where does MSM come from?

MSM is one of the three types of sulfur compounds that make up the majority (85 percent) of the sulfur found in all living things. The other two are DMSO (dimethylsulfoxide) and DMS (dimethylsulfide). The lives of these closely related compounds begin deep in the ocean, where a microscopic plant called Emiliana huxleyii grows and releases sulfur compounds called dimethylsulfonium salts. These salts transform into DMS, which then rises to the ocean's surface and enters the Earth's atmosphere. When DMS meets ozone and ultraviolet light in the upper atmosphere, it is converted into DMSO and MSM.

How does MSM get from the upper atmosphere to me?

As clouds move over the land, DMSO and MSM are attracted to them and dissolve. The DMSO and MSM mix with the moisture in the clouds and return to the Earth in rain droplets. Both compounds are absorbed by the plants through their roots, and the plants then concentrate the DMSO and MSM until they are up to 100 times their original strength. Over time, MSM becomes the primary bioavailable sulfur in the plants, which are then eaten by both animals and humans.

Sulfur is beneficial only if it is made accessible, or bioavailable, to the body. Eating the elemental mineral sulfur won't provide any health benefits. Instead, you must consume a form of sulfur that your body can assimilate. Plants take elemental sulfur from the soil and rainwater and convert it into one of several amino acids, which are then passed along to the animals, including humans, that eat them. These amino acids contain a bioavailable version of the mineral that can foster health in both the humans and animals that make plants a part of their diet.

And MSM is the form of sulfur my body needs?

Yes. MSM is a bioavailable form of sulfur that is found naturally in vegetables, legumes, and whole grains, as well as in animal protein foods such as milk, meat, poultry, and eggs. But MSM is a delicate structure and can be destroyed readily during food processing and cooking. MSM is found most reliably in foods that are completely unprocessed and uncooked, which means that most people aren't getting enough—unless they eat uncooked meat and eggs, unpasteurized milk, and unwashed produce; or their diet consists of all organic foods: fruits, vegetables, whole grains, soy products, and legumes. (In addition, overuse of agricultural soils has depleted their natural sulfur levels, meaning the crops that are grown and the animals that feed on them are not getting a sufficient amount of sulfur.)

How can I get enough MSM?

This is how supplemental MSM can help. Sold as a colorless, flavorless, and odorless white powder, packaged in capsules, crystals, or liquid, or blended into topical creams, gels, lotions, or a spray, MSM provides the body with the sulfur it needs, in a form it can use. When taken as directed, MSM is safe—no significant ill effects have been reported, and scientists know that as a water-soluble micronutrient, MSM will simply be eliminated from the body if it's not needed.

How important is MSM to my health?

Most people don't know that sulfur is very important to human health. Its role in the human body is essential enough to warrant it being considered an essential nutrient, or more precisely, an essential micronutrient. Sulfur also has a long history of external use, particularly in baths, poultices, and other applications to treat aches and pains. The role of sulfur in human health is explored in depth in chapter 2.

What is a micronutrient?

Scientist and nutritionists have a name for the things the body requires but that it can't make for itself: essential nutrients. Nutrients are divided into two categories: macronutrients, which are the things the body must get in large quantities, like protein, carbohydrates, and fat; and micronutrients, such as vitamins and minerals, which it requires in much smaller doses. Micronutrient minerals are, in turn, divided into two classes: major and trace. Major minerals, such as calcium, are measured in milligrams. Trace minerals are measured in micrograms, which are one-tenth the size of milligrams.

Micronutrients sound so insignificant; do we really need them?

Although we need only a minute amount of micronutrients, they are extremely important. Insufficient amounts of any micronutrient can lead to deficiency diseases; one of the best known is scurvy, brought on by chronic low levels of vitamin C.

However, scientists now know that even a slight deficiency in trace minerals can cause problems. And as scientists learn more and more about the delicate synergy of micronutrient actions within the body, they are able to pinpoint more reliably the exact compounds that are missing from our daily meals—and to add them in sufficient quantities to improve overall health and to foster specific benefits, such as pain relief. Thus we may well be entering an age in which nutrition is used to foster overall health and prevent disease—leaving behind much of our dependence on drugs that combat illnesses only after they've established themselves.

Dietary sulfur—or more specifically, MSM—falls into the category of the micronutrients known as trace minerals. Sulfur is included in the government's list of essential minerals, but it has not yet been assigned a Recommended Dietary Allowance (RDA).

How important is MSM for the body?

MSM is essential for several important bodily processes. Without enough MSM, you can develop serious deficiency problems. But with sufficient MSM, your body can function smoothly and you'll even be able to prevent or reverse many health problems.

Here's how it works. Your body uses MSM to build blood proteins and amino acids, as well as collagen and keratin, which are critical components of skin and connective tissue. Without MSM, you would literally fall apart, with no way to create the bonds that hold your cells and tissues together.

You also need MSM to produce insulin, a critical component in glucose metabolism and the key to preventing diabetes. MSM is also essential for maintaining healthy liver function and the proper acid/alkaline balance in the blood and internal organs, which, among other things, are absolutely essential to allow the body to detoxify itself properly through the digestive and circulatory systems. Equally important, minerals like MSM serve as catalysts for the actions of vitamins and other micronutrients. Without sulfur, essentials like vitamin C and the B vitamins can't do their jobs correctly. Ineffective synthesis of these vitamins can lead to even more health problems, not the least of which is a compromised immune system.

Another important function of MSM is the improvement of cell permeability throughout the body. It improves the ability of cells to pass nutrients along to other cells, creating many important health effects. Taking MSM means that cell membranes become more flexible, which translates into improved circulation and mobility, as well as quicker recovery times from muscle injuries. It also means that MSM can improve the absorption of other nutrients that you take in, including essential vitamins as well as other nutritional substances.

As you can see, a shortfall of MSM can spell disaster for your entire body, with troubles ranging from failing joints, diabetes, and chronic infections to poor healing and persistent swelling. Taking supplemental MSM can turn those problems around: relieve pain and inflammation, improve overall immunity, and bolster the body's ability to heal itself wherever it's needed.

I've heard many people talk about taking MSM for arthritis. How is MSM used to treat arthritis?

Perhaps the most exciting part of the MSM story is its ability to alleviate the pain and inflammation of arthritis, one of the most prevalent diseases in the world today, and, at least until recently, almost a foregone conclusion for anyone over 50.

MSM appears to aid the body in several functions that are necessary to prevent the development of arthritis—namely, to prevent the inflammation and irritation in the joints that cause pain, stiffness, and eventual deformity. MSM has been shown to relieve the pain and swelling of both osteoarthritis and rheumatoid arthritis, offering patients a new chance at life without painkillers—and without the grim prognosis so often heard from doctors that a condition will only get worse as the years go by. In fact, when combined with other natural approaches, MSM offers a real alternative to pharmaceutical pain relievers, and can even help to reverse the degenerative effects of arthritis. Thus, it has the potential to restore mobility and quality of life to the more than 40 million Americans now suffering from the disease.

I read about a new class of drugs for arthritis called super aspirins. How is MSM different from these new medications?

One of the most important differences between MSM and any drug, including super aspirins, is that MSM is a natural substance, a mineral that appears naturally in your body. That means it belongs in your body and has critical tasks to perform for your health and well-being. Super aspirins (which are explained in depth in chapter 4) are synthetically produced foreign substances, which is a main reason they, like other conventional drugs, cause side effects. Both MSM and super aspirins can relieve the pain and inflammation associated with arthritis, but they do it in different ways. MSM works to correct the cause of the pain and swelling, which in turn allows the body to heal itself and relieve these symptoms; super aspirins block the action of substances that cause pain and inflammation but do nothing to correct their cause.

What can I learn about MSM in this book?

MSM is rapidly emerging as one of the most promising health-care developments of its time. But as you'll soon discover, the story of MSM is still unfolding. As you read this book, you'll learn the latest information about MSM: theories as to how and why it works in the body; evidence from laboratory tests, clinical trials, and real-life applications; and areas of ongoing research that will no doubt give us even more information on the importance of maintaining adequate levels of sulfur in the body.

You'll hear from researchers who have tested MSM in their laboratories, plus doctors and nutritionists who have incorporated MSM into their practices. You'll also read what some patients have to say about how MSM has helped them treat osteoarthritis, rheumatoid arthritis, and a host of other medical problems.

Nearly as important as knowing more about what works for arthritis is identifying those remedies that are ineffective or those that can harm you. Products in these categories fall into several groups, including painkillers (analgesics) and anti-inflammatories, and the newest group, super aspirins. The pros and cons of using these drugs are explained. Ultimately, the decision about which remedies to use should be made by you and your health-care practitioner.

In addition, you'll also learn how you can put MSM to work for you: how to use oral and topical supplements, how much to use, safety information, and how to combine them with other natural treatments, including a ginger extract product called Zinaxin HMP-33. And you'll get a glimpse at the research that's going on right now, which is showing even broader applications for this remarkable substance.

Finally, you'll discover how MSM is also being used and researched for its effects on other health problems. Learn how people have gotten relief from allergies, scleroderma, parasite-related conditions, constipation, snoring, gastro-intestinal problems, heartburn, and various skin conditions from using MSM.

TWO

DMSO: Where It All Began

Sulfur is everywhere around us. It's near volcanoes and in garlic; it's in fungicides and on the moon. It falls to the earth dissolved in raindrops and lurks deep in the ocean. Sulfur is the sixteenth most abundant element in the Earth's crust. It exists in both a free form (also called elemental sulfur) and combined with other substances, as it is in pumice stone and gypsum. Elemental sulfur is used in industry to make products such as rubber and gunpowder, and in agriculture to make fungicides.

When it comes to health, sulfur is essential because it's in each and every cell in the body. Sulfur is especially prevalent in hair, nails, and skin. If you've ever burned a strand of your hair, the odor you smelled is sulfur. In fact, sulfur is the eighth most prevalent element in the body. The body, however, cannot use elemental sulfur. It can assimilate and use only the dietary form of sulfur called MSM.

Scientists have been aware that sulfur, in the form of MSM, is found in some of the amino acids that make up the protein in the food we eat. But its presence in protein foods was not enough to excite scientists to single out this nutrient as something special. Although scientists have long been interested in and studied other minerals such as calcium and iron, it wasn't until recently that researchers began to notice sulfur, and then only in passing. That is, until a combination of horse sense, serendipity, and persistence brought MSM into the forefront.

To appreciate why sulfur came into the spotlight, let's learn when and how interest in this mineral originated. In the early 1960s, Robert Herschler, M.D., and Stanley W. Jacob, M.D., began to explore the therapeutic possibilities of a compound called DMSO, or dimethylsulfoxide. This compound was found to be effective in relieving inflammation, osteoarthritis, rheumatoid arthritis, gout, burns, interstitial cystitis, and various viral, bacterial, fungal, and parasitic skin infections. Approximately 100,000 people received DMSO during clinical trials, and the results were very promising.

During the early days of studying DMSO, Drs. Jacob and Herschler also teamed up with Dr. John Metcalf, an equine veterinarian in Auburn, Washington. They experimented with administering DMSO to horses and discovered that it reduced inflammation, promoted circulation, cleared up lung problems, and healed wounds and lacerations. Topical application of DMSO eliminated inflammation of injured joints and limbs and resolved lameness.

By 1965, Drs. Jacob and Herschler had evidence that DMSO helped both people and animals. In that same year, people lost the choice of whether they could take DMSO at all when the Food and Drug Administration ordered that the substance no longer be given to humans. This decision had nothing to do with the one side effect people found most bothersome about DMSO: the odor. Everyone who takes DMSO, including animals, emits a fishlike odor and has a fishlike taste in his mouth that lasts the entire time he takes the supplement. (Flatulence, too, is often a problem.) Instead, the ban was mandated because there were findings of eye damage in rabbits, pigs, and dogs that had DMSO administered into their eyes. Although no problems were observed in human eyes, the ban remained in effect until 1978, when the FDA approved DMSO for use in humans for one disorder only—

interstitial cystitis, a painful inflammatory disease of the bladder that usually affects middle-aged women.

Because MSM is a byproduct of DMSO, does it have the same "fishy" odor that DMSO has?

No. When DMSO enters the body, in any form, it breaks down into several components. One is DMS, or dimethylsulfide, which is responsible for the fishlike odor and taste, as well as the flatulence. Another component is MSM, which does not have these properties.

Do where does MSM fit into the DMSO story?

In the meantime, Dr. Herschler, who had been researching DMSO on his own since the late 1950s, in 1975 began studying a metabolite of DMSO called methysulfonylmethane, or MSM. His research suggested that it was the MSM that gave the DMSO its healing abilities. When Dr. Herschler discovered that MSM had the ability to soften skin, he and Dr. Jacob investigated the use of MSM in people with scleroderma, a disease in which the skin and various organs lose their elasticity and in some cases eventually causes death.

The patients treated with topical MSM improved, but the doctors still needed to determine whether MSM was toxic. After toxicity tests, which involve placing irritants into rabbits' eyes, showed MSM to be nontoxic, Dr. Herschler took testing one step further and treated irritated rabbit eyes with MSM. To his surprise, the MSM eliminated the irritation. Now the researchers knew they had a substance that was nontoxic, an anti-inflammatory, and which could revive skin elasticity.

Only after years of controversy did the FDA allow scientists to resume clinical trials with DMSO in 1980. The flurry of activity that followed the FDA's decision to allow trials included research by Drs. Jacob and Herschler, who found that when DMSO is heated, it crystallizes and leaves behind 99.9 percent MSM, or sulfur. In 1983, the researchers predicted that "this [MSM] will receive international attention as a dietary supplement." Drs. Jacob and Herschler were excited because their research suggested "that a minimum concentration in the body may be critical to both normal function and structure." It was then their task to uncover what those essential functions were.

What vital functions does sulfur perform in the body?

Nearly all the body's tissues contain MSM, the biological (organic) form of sulfur, particularly those that consist of a high percentage of protein. Sulfur has the critical task of holding together the molecular structure of proteins, which are composed of amino acids—the building blocks of protein. Without sulfur, proteins would fall apart. Of all the amino acids, the ones that contain sulfur in their chemical framework are cystine, cysteine, methionine, and taurine. These are known as the sulfur amino acids.

The main purpose of sulfur is to lend strength, shape, and hardness to the structures it inhabits. Approximately 50 percent of the 100 mg of sulfur in the body is concentrated in the muscles, bones, and skin. Two types of protein that contain high levels of sulfur are collagen, which is found in bones, connective tissue, and teeth; and keratin, found in nails, skin, and hair. Sufficient levels of sulfur in collagen and keratin help keep your bones, teeth, and nails hard; your skin blemish-free; your muscles flexible; your connective tissues intact; and your hair shiny and thick. Without enough sulfur, none of these structures, and even many more, would not heal and repair properly. (For details about specific medical conditions that respond to MSM, see chapter 9.)

What other health benefits does sulfur provide?

Sulfur is involved in nearly every part of the body's functioning. (A detailed discussion of how sulfur is used to treat numerous medical conditions and symptoms is presented in chapter 9.) For example, sulfur is an indispensable factor in the functioning of B vitamin biotin, which helps metabolize fat and facilitate cell growth. Among people who have diabetes, sulfur is especially critical because it aids in carbohydrate metabolism and the utilization of glucose. (See "Diabetes" in chapter 9.)

The B vitamin thiamine (B_1) also has a sulfur component. Thiamine helps convert sugars and starch into energy, boosts blood circulation, and stimulates digestion. It is a necessary factor in the formation of blood, in the maintenance of heart and intestinal muscle, and as a protective agent against the damaging effects of excess smoking and alcohol.

Sulfur stimulates the production of bile acids, which are instrumental in the digestion and absorption of fat. It also performs a balancing act by maintaining the body's pH (acid/alkaline) levels. Its ability to control acidity in the stomach can help prevent ulcers and heartburn.

Muscles and tissues benefit from sulfur's ability to reduce inflammation, which can limit mobility and cause pain. Sulfur also reduces muscle spasms and cramps.

Your mental and emotional states even benefit from sulfur, as it promotes mental calmness and increases alertness and the ability to concentrate. The immune system gets a boost from sulfur, and the ability of the body to heal wounds and repair damaged cells is enhanced.

Yet another benefit of MSM may come from eating foods that contain sulfur, especially vegetables such as broccoli, cabbage, kale, leeks, horscradish, onion, cauliflower, daikon, brussels sprouts, and kohlrabi. In addition to supplying sulfur, these particular foods have cancer-inhibiting abilities.

What happens if I don't get enough sulfur?

Without sufficient sulfur, blood does not clot well, cells don't utilize oxygen properly, insulin can't be produced, and several vital enzymes will malfunction. The result over time can be increased susceptibility to illness and disease, fatigue, and tissue and organ malfunction. Sulfur also protects against the harmful effects of pollution and radiation, which makes it useful in slowing down the aging process.

It does not appear that people with a sulfur deficiency suffer from any specific disease caused directly by inadequate levels of the nutrient. However, protein is the main dietary source of sulfur; thus a diet low in protein will be accompanied by insufficient sulfur, evident by low levels of the sulfur amino acids. The synergistic relationship among sulfur and the various nutrients mentioned above demonstrates the importance of maintaining a sufficient level of sulfur in your diet.

Although protein deficiency is generally not a problem in the United States, the elderly are especially prone to it. These individuals often do not consume a nutritious diet because of poor health, inadequate income, or social isolation, or because they have a poor appetite due to illness or medication use. Supplementation with MSM can not only eliminate sulfur deficiency in the elderly, but can also have a positive effect on medical problems that often afflict them, especially osteoarthritis, rheumatoid arthritis, and constipation.

What are some signs of sulfur deficiency?

Scientists estimate that the body uses up to ⅛ teaspoon of MSM per day. Your body has several external ways to let you know when your sulfur levels are low. If your body is low on sulfur and vitamin C, you may notice that wounds such as cuts, scrapes, and burns do not heal well and leave a raised scar. Dry skin is a symptom of biotin deficiency, as are hair loss, brittle hair, and fragile nails. Nails are composed of 98 percent keratin, which has a high sulfur content. If your nails are soft or brittle and you are consuming sufficient vitamin A and vitamin E (10,000–15,000 IU beta-carotene [vitamin A] and 400 IU vitamin E), chances are your sulfur intake is low.

Although not specific signs of a deficiency of MSM, some physical and medical problems are aggravated by low levels of this nutrient. If you have any of the following conditions, MSM supplementation may help: arthritis, allergies, Alzheimer's disease, candida infection, chronic fatigue, diabetes, diverticulosis, hair loss, high cholesterol levels, migraines, scar tissue, soft or brittle nails, sore muscles and joints, ulcers, and wrinkles. Many of these health problems are discussed in detail in chapter 9.

How important to my health are sulfur amino acids?

Of the four sulfur amino acids, three are classified as nonessential, which means the body manufactures them. Only methionine is essential, which means it must be taken in, preferably through diet, or through supplements. The existence of cysteine, cystine, and taurine depend on methionine, because each of these three amino acids are directly or indirectly created from it. Taurine is synthesized from methionine throughout the body and from cysteine in the liver; the body converts methionine into cysteine; and cystine is the result of the oxidation and bonding of two cysteine molecules. Thus insufficient methionine can have a devastating effect on the other three sulfur amino acids.

Methionine is needed by the body to break down fat and help prevent fat buildup in the liver and arteries. Adequate levels of methionine are also necessary to maintain muscle strength and promote the excretion of estrogen. Some studies suggest that methionine may help prevent formation of kidney stones. Toxic agents such as mercury, arsenic, and lead are eliminated from the body with the help of methionine. A deficiency of both methionine and taurine is associated with certain allergies and with autoimmune disease.

A deficiency of cysteine automatically results in a lack of cystine because the latter is created when two cysteines bond together. Because cysteine is found in keratin, a deficiency of this amino acid may appear as soft nails, lackluster hair, and poor skin elasticity. Some psychotic patients have been found to have low levels of cysteine.

Taurine is viewed as a conditionally essential amino acid because it appears to be essential only in infants and not adults. Low levels of taurine have been linked to depression, hypertension, kidney failure, and hypothyroidism. Recommended supplementation levels needed to correct these conditions range from 500 mg to 5,000 mg.

Which foods are good sources of sulfur?

Sulfur is found in significant amounts in whole grains, legumes, mustard, onions, garlic, asparagus, cabbage, brussels sprouts, broccoli, red peppers, milk, and eggs. Specific sources for methionine include sunflower seeds (exceptionally high), beans and soybeans, lentils, onions, garlic, yogurt, eggs, and fish. Cysteine is found in garlic, onions, yogurt, and wheat germ. Taurine is found only in animal proteins, yet because the body synthesizes taurine from methionine, vegetarians usually have no problem with taurine deficiency if they eat foods that contain methionine. Theoretically it is possible to get all the sulfur you need from your diet, but few people do.

Why is it hard to get sulfur from food?

At one time, fruits, vegetables, grains, and other foods were grown without the use of pesticides and herbicides. The rain was free of pollutants. Milk and other dairy products were produced without hormones, steroids, and other additives. Most food was free of artificial colors, flavors, stabilizers, texturizers, and other chemicals. For the most part, food was picked fresh and consumed fresh, or preserved in a natural way. Times have changed.

Today most of our food is preserved, packaged, and riddled with chemicals. Although there are growing numbers of organic foods on the market, the majority of Americans still consume a diet that is dominated by processed food, much of it devoid of nutrients, including sulfur, but rich in fat, cholesterol, and toxins. Conventionally grown produce is harvested from soil that has been stripped of its nutritional value through over-farming, use of toxic chemicals, and inadequate rejuvenation of the soil. What little nutritional value there is in the food is then removed or destroyed during the sequence of harvesting, storing, shipping, processing, and packaging.

Thus unless you are very diligent about eating only organic foods and consuming a lot of fresh, raw foods, your intake of foods that should contain sulfur is probably not providing you with the sulfur you need.

What other reasons might I be sulfur deficient?

According to Marcellus Walker, M.D., a physician in Honesdale, Pennsylvania, who prescribes MSM to patients in his practice, many people are sulfur deficient because in addition to not getting enough sulfur from food, their bodies are toxic with heavy metals and other environmental toxins. Heavy metals, such as lead and mercury (found in amalgam dental fillings), and environmental toxins, such as second-hand smoke, chemical fumes, and water pollutants, deprive the body of sulfur.

How much sulfur does the body need each day?

Even though sulfur is an essential nutrient for health, no RDA has been established. Some researchers have estimated that the human body needs between 850 and 1,400 mg of sulfur per day to replace this nutrient's turnover in the body, depending on a person's size, age, gender, and dietary habits. Ideally, any diet that contains sufficient protein, including high-quality plant proteins, should have an adequate amount of sulfur. But as it was explained above, most foods in the standard American diet are sulfur-deficient. That fact has lead many health experts to suggest that Americans take a sulfur supplement, or MSM.

Why is MSM the best source of sulfur?

Sulfur is found in many different forms in nature, but the only form that the body can readily and easily use is the organic, dietary form known as MSM. Unlike DMSO, another form of sulfur that has been used for years around the world to treat many medical conditions, especially various types of pain, MSM is colorless and odorless and does not have adverse side effects. It has been used as a supplemental source of sulfur for years by tens of thousands of people with no reports of toxic or allergic reactions or intolerance, even at large doses.

Study after study has shown MSM to be non-allergic and nonpyretic (non–fever causing) and to combine easily and safely with other pharmaceutical substances. In fact, MSM actually prevents the body from overreacting to other medications. Because MSM is such a neutral substance, it is used as a blood diluent. Some researchers believe it can also be used as a safe way to deliver drugs to the body, although this use is under debate.

What about DMSO? Isn't that a source of sulfur, too?

DMSO, or dimethylsulfoxide, is an all-natural substance that is a by-product of the process used to make wood pulp. Like MSM, which is derived from DMSO, it contains sulfur and possesses the healing characteristics of the organic nutrient.

Yet DMSO has a few stumbling blocks around

its use, especially in the United States. Since it was first introduced to the medical world by Stanley W. Jacob, M.D., and his research team in 1963, it has been the subject of more than 11,000 research articles. Although countless studies show that it possesses anti-inflammatory and antioxidant abilities, the FDA still only allows one use in humans—treatment of interstitial cystitis (a painful inflammatory bladder disorder). Veterinary practitioners, however, are permitted to use it and have done so very successfully for decades for treatment of arthritis, connective tissue damage, skin disorders, and other medical conditions in dogs, horses, and other animals.

Outside the United States, DMSO is prescribed and used in more than 100 countries, especially for arthritis, as well as for muscle pain, athletic injuries, headache, skeletal disorders, and acute traumatic injuries. In Russia, for example, it is estimated that 50 percent of people with arthritic conditions take DMSO as part of their therapy. Fortunately, people in the United States can reap nearly all the benefits of DMSO (and none of the fishlike odor and taste, flatulence, and rare instances of skin irritation) by using MSM.

DMSO may have some advantages MSM does not. Although both substances pass easily through the skin and tissues, which helps make them effective in relieving pain and inflammation, there is debate as to whether MSM can transport medications into and through the body, a quality DMSO possesses. And although DMSO has antioxidant abilities, whether MSM has the same capabilities has not yet been proved.

❁
THREE
❁

Your Body, Your Cells, and MSM at Work

The human body is a fascinating, complex structure, composed of 70 trillion cells, all busily conducting their business. Those cells are composed of and utilize certain elements which are necessary for the body and all of its various systems to function properly. Four main elements make up the majority of the body's weight: oxygen, carbon, hydrogen, and nitrogen. Nine other elements combined nearly round out the remaining 4 percent, with yet another 11 trace components that do just that. Sulfur, or MSM, is one of the 9 elements, and comprises a mere 0.25 percent of the total body weight—a seemingly very insignificant factor in the total picture.

Yet MSM is a critical nutrient in the whole scheme of things. Simply put, without MSM, you could not exist. MSM, like all the other nutrients in the body, does not exist in a vacuum. Its presence affects dozens of other substances in the body, which in turn affect many others. Nearly every cell in your body contains some MSM, and each of those cells has a job which is designed to keep your body functioning at its optimal level.

In this chapter, you will learn about the synergistic relationship that exists between MSM and some of the other nutrients with which it interacts. This brief overview will give you a better understanding of how important MSM is to your health.

WHAT DO CELLS DO?

The body never sleeps. Even while you are enjoying a good night's snooze, your body's cells are busy reproducing, repairing, respiring, and performing other vital functions. To keep up the continuous schedule of building and maintenance, your body requires certain raw materials in the form of nutrients. Each nutrient has one or more essential tasks to do, and if one nutrient is deficient or lacking, the body cannot continue in an efficient manner. The result is cells that become either dysfunctional or irreparably damaged, which can lead to illness and disease.

What are cells?

Cells are complete, minute living units that are composed of a nucleus, cytoplasm, and a cell membrane. The nucleus contains the genetic material; the cytoplasm is composed of various organ-like structures called organelles, which perform functions such as respiration, excretion, and digestion; and the cell membrane allows the passage of nutrients and other materials both into and out of the cell.

The body is composed of many different types of cells; for example, nerve cells, blood cells (the only cells that do not have a nucleus), and muscle cells. Similar cells that group together form tissues, such as muscle tissue and connective tissue. As mentioned in chapter 2, MSM is a critical component in the formation of connective tissue and proteins.

What kind of nutrients do cells use?

Nutrients are substances needed by living cells to maintain their existence. Proteins, carbohydrates, fats, water, vitamins, and minerals are the main classifications of nutrients your cells need to perform their designated functions. Other terms you may have heard for nutrients, such as antioxidant, bioflavonoid, enzyme, phytonutrient, fatty acid, and amino acid, describe types of nutrients found within these main classifications. MSM is just one of many minerals that acts as a cofactor (a coworker, if you will), with other nutrients to maintain cell health.

What is the difference between vitamins and minerals?

Vitamins are organic substances which are essential to life. Because they cannot be synthesized in the body, they must be obtained from food, although a few vitamins are ingested in a provitamin form (called precursors) and are then converted into vitamins once in the body. One example is beta-carotene, which is converted into vitamin A once it is in the body.

Vitamins are considered to be micronutrients because they appear in relatively small amounts in the body when compared with the macronutrients—carbohydrates, proteins, fats, and water. The primary functions of vitamins are to regulate metabolism and to assist the chemical processes that release energy from food. Vitamins work along with enzymes (catalysts for the chemical reactions that occur in the body) as coenzymes to ensure that the body systems function properly.

Minerals are inorganic, naturally occurring substances that are found in the earth. Similar to vitamins, minerals also act as coenzymes in that they allow the body to properly perform its tasks. Those tasks include the blood and bone formation, body fluid maintenance, protein metabolism, energy production, nerve transmission, and muscle contraction. To accomplish these functions, minerals work in combination (as cofactors) with vitamins, enzymes, hormones, and other substances.

MSM AND YOUR CELLS

Once vitamins and minerals are absorbed into the body, they become part of the synergistic relationship that exists within each human being. This relationship works optimally when nutrients are in balance, which allows two or more nutrients to combine and work together to perform a specific task or function. One example of this is explained below, in which MSM and vitamin C cooperate to build and repair cells. Another example is the cooperation between MSM and magnesium, in which the two work to detoxify sulfuric acid and allow it to be excreted through the kidneys.

How does the body absorb MSM?

The body utilizes many different minerals, some of which are difficult to absorb. MSM, however, is an organic form of sulfur and is extremely well absorbed by the body. Most dietary sulfur is ingested in foods that contain one or more of the sulfur amino acids. About 75 percent of the amino acids are metabolized for the purpose of creating new proteins. The liver is the main site of amino acid metabolism. When you take any of the oral forms of MSM, some of the sulfur binds immediately to the mucosal membrane receptor sites, while the rest is absorbed quickly into the bloodstream. Even though MSM is easily absorbed, many people are sulfur deficient, for the reasons explained in chapter 2.

What does MSM do once it enters the body?

MSM is readily accepted by the body because it is a negatively charged molecule. This means that MSM molecules tend to give up electrons and pair up with other substances that are positively charged, especially toxic agents such as mercury and harmful bacteria. This tendency to find and adhere to potentially harmful substances is a critical part of one of the other important functions MSM performs: transportation. MSM allows the free passage of water and nutrients into the cells through the cell walls; and it allows toxins and cell waste to leave the cells. This transportation process is called osmosis, and without it, you could not survive. When osmosis is hindered by insufficient sulfur, the cell walls lose their flexibility. The result can be any number of medical problems or illnesses: for example, hardened arteries, sore muscles, hypoglycemia, high blood sugar, migraines, varicose veins, scar tissue, wrinkles, and damaged lung tissue.

MSM is also involved in the production of enzymes and hormones, including the hormone insulin. Both hormones and enzymes depend on a healthy supply of amino acids, the building blocks of protein in the body. All of the amino acids must bind with dietary sulfur in order to conduct these manufacturing processes, without which you could not exist. Because protein is the main component of most of the body's soft tissues, maintaining an adequate level of MSM is necessary for healthy muscles, tendons, ligaments, skin, and mucous membranes throughout the body.

Which nutrients are needed for MSM to be properly assimilated in the body?

Much research has been done on the interaction between nutrients and how they each affect their bioavailability. *Bioavailability* refers to the amount of an ingested nutrient that is absorbed and made available for the body's needs. Like all nutrients, MSM depends on adequate levels of specific vitamins and minerals to be assimilated and absorbed properly. (See following table for the Recommended Daily Allowances and Suggested Therapeutic Dosages of vitamins and minerals.)

RDA and Therapeutic Doses of Nutrients

Nutrient	RDA/EMDA*	Therapeutic Dosage
Vitamin A (retinol)	4,000–5,000 IU	5,000–10,000 IU
Beta-carotene	2.4–3 mg	5,000–25,000 IU
Vitamin D	400 IU	100–400 IU
Vitamin E (d-alpha tocopherol)	400 IU	400–1,200 IU
Vitamin K	65–80 mcg	60–900 mcg
Vitamin C	60 mg	500–9,000 mg
Vitamin B_1 (thiamin)	1.1–1.5 mg	10–100 mg
Vitamin B_2 (riboflavin)	1.3–1.7 mg	10–100 mg
Vitamin B_6 (pyridoxine)	1.6–2 mg	25–100 mg
Niacin	15–19 mg	10–100 mg
Biotin	30–100 mcg	100–300 mcg
Pantothenic acid	4–7 mg	25–100 mg
Folic acid	400 mcg	400–1,000 mcg
Vitamin B_{12}	2–2.2 mcg	200–1,000 mcg
Boron	1–2 mg	1–6 mg
Calcium	800–1,500 mg	250–750 mg
Chromium	50–200 mcg	200–400 mcg
Copper	1.5–3 mg	1–2 mg
Iodine	150 mcg	50–150 mcg
Iron	10 mg	15–30 mg
Magnesium	280–350 mg	250–500 mg
Manganese	2.5–5 mg	10–15 mg
Molybdenum	150–500 mcg	10–25 mcg

Nutrient	RDA/EMDA*	Therapeutic Dosage
Potassium	3,500 mg	200–500 mg
Selenium	55–70 mcg	100–200 mcg
Zinc	15–30 mg	15–45 mg

*Therapeutic doses support optimal health and/or treat specific conditions. Nutrients that have not been assigned an RDA have been given an EDMR, or Estimated Daily Minimum Requirement.

Those nutrients include biotin (one of the B vitamins), pantothenic acid (vitamin B_5), potassium, and thiamine (vitamin B_1). Likewise, each one of these nutrients depends on others for its ability to be assimilated: biotin needs folic acid (another B vitamin) and pantothenic acid; pantothenic acid needs the B-complex vitamins and vitamins A, C, and E; and so on. This cooperative relationship demonstrates the importance of maintaining a balance of vitamins, minerals, and other nutrients in the body.

What role does MSM play in building and repairing cells?

MSM works side by side with vitamins and amino acids as building material for the creation of new cells and repairing damaged ones. During the manufacturing process, the body constantly draws upon its supply of vitamin C. As a water soluble vitamin (one that cannot be stored in the body and is excreted within one to four days), vitamin C needs to be replaced daily. MSM also is depleted rapidly and needs daily replacement. If either of these building materials is absent or low, the manufacturing and repairing processes suffer.

Many people are taking MSM to relieve pain and inflammation. How does MSM accomplish this?

Most of the nerve cells responsible for sensing pain are located in the soft tissues of the body. When there is a shift or change in the pressure inside the cells versus that outside the cells, pain can result.

An example of this phenomenon occurs among some people who have arthritis. When a rainstorm is approaching, the barometric pressure drops. This results in a decline in pressure outside the body's cells, which causes the cells to swell because the pressure inside the cells is greater. The result is pain and inflammation, if the walls of the tissue cells lack flexibility and permeability. Taking MSM supplements can make the cell walls flexible and allow fluids to pass through the cell walls and tissues more easily. Once the fluids are allowed to flow more readily, any change in pressure outside the cells can be compensated for by the exchange of fluids through the membrane, which in turn can eliminate or significantly reduce pain and inflammation.

MSM also helps reduce pain and inflammation by promoting blood circulation, which stimulates healing, and by reducing muscle spasm.

You can also take MSM for pain relief by applying it topically to the area that is painful and inflamed. For this purpose, MSM is available as a lotion, a gel, and a spray mist.

What types of pain can be treated successfully with MSM?

In addition to arthritis (which is discussed in depth in chapter 5), MSM has been effective in the treatment of back pain, dental pain, burns, bruises, tendinitis, bursitis, carpel tunnel syndrome, headache, menstrual cramps, leg pain (associated with restless leg syndrome), migraine, and temporal mandibular joint (TMJ) dysfunction.

FOUR

*What You Need to Know About
Super Aspirin and Other
Conventional Arthritis Remedies*

Before you make the decision whether or not to
take MSM for arthritis, you need to know what
other treatment options are available to you and
understand the pros and cons of using them.
Every day, millions of Americans ingest one or
more various prescription or over-the-counter
drugs with the hope that they will relieve or
eliminate the pain, inflammation, and loss of mobility associated with their arthritis. These compounds have familiar names, and some not so
familiar—aspirin, ibuprofen, sulindac, naproxen
—and fall into two of several categories of
medications routinely used to treat arthritis:
analgesics (painkillers) and nonsteroidal anti-
inflammatory drugs (NSAIDs). One common
habit of people with arthritis is that they

often take one or more of these drugs every day and over a long period of time. Depending on an individual's susceptibility to chemical agents and his or her medical condition, even occasional use of these drugs can cause troublesome or even serious side effects or interactions. That's because these drugs are powerful foreign bodies, designed to kill pain, and in the process they create toxic reactions in the body and actually hinder healing.

As the millennium draws to a close, a new category of drugs is hitting the market. Labeled "super aspirins," these drugs, which include Celebrex and Vioxx, are designed to provide the relief offered by the drugs traditionally used to treat arthritis, but without the adverse effects associated with the older medications. This chapter explores both the "old" arthritis treatments and the new, including a description of what they are, how they work, and the problems they can cause.

NONSTEROIDAL ANTI-INFLAMMATORY DRUGS

Nonsteroidal anti-inflammatory drugs (NSAIDs) are among the most commonly used drugs in the world. In 1997, 77 million prescriptions for

NSAIDs were written in the United States alone, and sales of NSAIDs reached $8 billion. Approximately 33 million Americans take NSAIDs regularly. The drugs in this category are often used to treat pain, arthritis, headache, fever, and menstrual cramps and include the oldest and perhaps best known drug, aspirin. Nonsteroidal anti-inflammatory drugs work by blocking enzymes known collectively as cyclooxygenase (COX). Cyclooxygenase is necessary for the production of prostaglandins, which are substances that cause inflammation. Inflammation is accompanied by pain, heat, redness, and swelling, the hallmarks of arthritis. NSAIDs block the action of two types of COX enzymes: COX-1, which helps protect the stomach lining against irritation from the drugs; and COX-2, which causes pain and inflammation. Thus NSAIDs are wolves in sheep's clothing: they inhibit pain and swelling, but also prevent the stomach protection offered by COX-1.

In addition to aspirin, other NSAIDs available either over the counter or by prescription include diclofenac, diflunisal, etodolac, fenoprofen, floctafenine, flurbiprofen, ibuprofen, indomethacin, ketoprofen, ketorolac, meclofenamate, mefenamic acid, nabumetone, naproxen, oxaprozin, phenylbutazone, piroxicam, sulindac, tenoxicam, tiaprofenic acid, and tolmetin.

What's the difference between aspirin and an NSAID? Are they the same?

Aspirin and other NSAIDs are often prescribed by physicians to treat most types of arthritis. Aspirin, which is also referred to as acetylsalicylic acid, or ASA, helps relieve mild to moderate pain and inflammation. If your arthritis symptoms fall into this category, and you do not experience the stomach and intestinal irritation aspirin often causes, aspirin may be sufficient for you. If you have chronic or more severe symptoms, it may be necessary to take high doses of aspirin—600 to 900 mg or more up to four times a day—in order to get relief from arthritis. In such cases, your physician may recommend you take one of the other NSAIDs. Nonsteroidal anti-inflammatory drugs work like aspirin but are generally more potent and longer lasting, and they have less severe side effects. Some are available over the counter; others are available by prescription only.

What side effects does aspirin cause?

The main side effect associated with the use of aspirin is stomach irritation, which can lead to bleeding and ulceration in the stomach. Other problems include ringing in the ears, dizziness, and reduced hearing. The chance of experiencing these symptoms increases the more aspirin you take. High doses of aspirin (12 or more tablets per day) can cause your body to both excrete greater amounts of vitamin C and absorb less of it; to lose iron through bleeding in the gastrointestinal tract; and to decrease in blood levels of folic acid.

What are the side effects of NSAIDs?

Like aspirin, the number one side effect of NSAIDs is stomach irritation. Other common adverse reactions include nausea, stomach cramps, headache, diarrhea, rash, and bleeding from the rectum (if using suppositories). Less common are drowsiness, vomiting, gaseousness, dry mouth, tremors, insomnia, and depression. Problems with a drop in blood pressure and reduced kidney function may occur among people who are older than 60 or who have heart disease, kidney disease, or peptic ulcer. Prolonged use of NSAIDs is associated with eye damage, abnormal liver function, and kidney problems.

The side effects caused by NSAIDs is serious business. According to the *Journal of Rheumatology* (18 [suppl. 28], 1991), NSAIDs are responsible for more than 76,000 hospitalizations and 7,600 deaths each year in the United States.

Is it possible to be allergic to aspirin and other NSAIDs?

Some people do have an allergic reaction to aspirin and other NSAIDs. If you experience wheezing, difficulty breathing, rash, hives, itching, puffy eyelids, or nasal polyps soon after taking NSAIDs, you are likely having an allergic reaction. Call 911 or go to a hospital emergency department immediately.

Do NSAIDs react with food, alcohol, or other medications I may be taking?

Nonsteroidal anti-inflammatory drugs generally do not interact negatively with food. In fact, it is recommended that you take them with food to help reduce stomach irritation. If, however, you are taking other medications, NSAIDs may cause problems. Because there is an increased risk of bleeding associated with the use of NSAIDs and oral anticoagulants (drugs that prevent blood clots—e.g., warfarin sodium) or cephalosporins, do not take these drugs together with NSAIDs unless under the direct supervision of your physician. Taking thyroid hormones and NSAIDs can cause rapid heartbeat and a rise in blood pressure. If you take two or more NSAIDs together, including aspirin and another NSAID, you significantly increase your risk of stomach ulcer and stomach bleeding. Consult with your physician before you start any new medications.

I've experienced stomach distress when taking NSAIDs. Will acetaminophen help relieve my arthritis symptoms?

Acetaminophen is often used by people who are allergic to aspirin, who have peptic ulcer, or who need pain relief from osteoarthritis. This analgesic relieves mild to moderate pain and fever but has no effect on inflammation or stiffness. For this reason, some people take both acetaminophen and an NSAID with the hope that the combination will provide greater pain relief. This is a dangerous mixture, however, and over time may lead to kidney disease. Acetaminophen rarely causes side effects but should be avoided if you have kidney disease or liver damage.

OTHER ARTHRITIS REMEDIES

Analgesics and NSAIDs are the most common treatments for osteoarthritis and rheumatoid arthritis and the easiest to obtain, as most can be purchased over the counter. For patients with long-term or severe disease, which often significantly limits their ability to function, other types of drugs are often prescribed. These include disease-modifying anti-rheumatic drugs (DMARDs) for people with rheumatoid arthritis, and corticosteroids for patients with either osteoarthritis or rheumatoid arthritis.

What are disease-modifying anti-rheumatic drugs?

Drugs in this category are designed to reduce the symptoms of rheumatoid arthritis, lupus, and some other forms of arthritis, as well as limit progression of the disease. They are more potent than NSAIDs but are slower acting. These drugs are rarely taken alone; NSAIDs are typically prescribed and sometimes corticosteroids at low doses are also given. Some of the more commonly prescribed DMARDs include hydroxychloroquine, gold, and methotrexate.

My doctor wants to give me hydroxychloroquine. What is it and what can it do for my arthritis?

This DMARD was originally developed to treat malaria, but it has been effective in reducing the inflammation, swelling, stiffness, and joint pain of rheumatoid arthritis and lupus. It also helps prevent disease progression. Unlike most other DMARDs, hydroxychloroquine does not suppress the immune system.

What side effects does hydroxychloroquine cause?

Hydroxychloroquine use can cause vomiting, nausea, dizziness, loss of appetite, rash, itching, headache, bitter taste in the mouth, and diarrhea. In rare cases, prolonged use can cause damage to the retina of the eye. Anyone who takes hydroxychloroquine should have routine eye examinations, every six to nine months, while taking the drug.

What is methotrexate?

This DMARD is widely prescribed for rheumatoid arthritis. It reduces the activity and progression of this arthritis form as well as some other arthritic conditions such as psoriatic arthritis. It works by changing the way the body uses folic acid, a vitamin that is essential for cell growth. It is often prescribed along with NSAIDs and prednisone.

Methotrexate is usually taken once a week, either by injection or by mouth. It generally takes three weeks or longer before relief is apparent.

What are the side effects of methotrexate?

Common side effects include nausea, vomiting, loss of appetite, diarrhea, mouth sores, and stomach upset. Some people get relief from these side effects by taking supplements of folic acid.

More serious and less common adverse reactions include liver damage and lung damage, which shows as shortness of breath, fever, or a cough which taking methotrexate. If you take methotrexate, you will be required to undergo routine laboratory testing every one to two months to monitor any changes in your bone marrow and liver.

How effective is gold therapy?

Gold treatments are used for people with rheumatoid arthritis, juvenile rheumatoid arthritis, and psoriatic arthritis. It is usually most effective when given to people in the early stages of their disease, although it can provide good relief for individuals in any stage. The exact reason why it works is still unknown.

Physicians generally prescribe gold therapy if other treatments, including aspirin, NSAIDs, and prednisone, have not been successful. About 50 percent of people treated with gold experience improvement. This DMARD does work slowly, however; most patients do not experience a decrease in joint pain, swelling, or stiffness until 2 to 6 months after starting treatment. Treatments can be given either by injection directly into a muscle or taken in capsule form. Gold treatments generally lose their effectiveness after 2 to 3 years.

What are the side effects of gold treatment?

The most common side effect of oral gold treatment is diarrhea. Those associated with injectable treatment include rash, mouth sores, low white blood count, and a metallic taste in the mouth. All of these reactions can persist for months after stopping treatment. Serious side effects include damage to the liver, intestines, and lungs.

What are corticosteroids?

Corticosteroids or glucocorticoids are drugs used to treat the inflammation associated with diseases such as arthritis and lupus and thus help reduce the amount of damage to the joints and organs. These drugs, which include cortisone, dexamethasone, hydrocortone, prednisolone, and prednisone, among others, are not the same as anabolic steroids, which are used and abused by some athletes. Corticosteroids are not without adverse effects, however, and their use should be carefully monitored by a doctor.

What are the common side effects associated with corticosteroid use?

The severity and frequency of side effects caused by corticosteroid use is related to the dose. High doses of the drugs can cause significant weight gain in the form of both water retention and body fat. They can also increase your appetite, which can further contribute to a weight increase.

Mood swings can occur at both low and high dosages, although they are more likely to occur at high doses. Some people experience bouts of nervousness, insomnia, psychosis, weakness in the leg and arm muscles, blurred vision, acne, round face (also known as moon face), osteoporosis, thinning hair, excessive hair growth, and slow wound healing. In most cases, these symptoms appear after a few weeks of taking a high dose of corticosteroids.

Corticosteroids also damage your nutritional state by decreasing absorption of vitamin D and causing you to quickly lose zinc, potassium, and vitamin C, which can lead to deficiencies. You may want to take therapeutic dosages of these supplements if you take corticosteroids (see table on pages 44–45).

Can corticosteroids cause serious or life-threatening side effects?

After using high doses of corticosteroids for a few weeks or months, some people develop high blood pressure, stomach ulcers, high blood sugar, and stomach irritation. Anyone who has existing diabetes, hypertension, or ulcers needs to discuss his or her medical history with a doctor before starting treatment. Another serious problem with corticosteroids is that they are immunosuppressives, which means they depress the ability of the immune system to fight off infection. Depending on the state of a person's immune system, use of corticosteroids can result in infection.

Less common side effects associated with moderate or long-term use of corticosteroids include glaucoma, severe muscle weakness, and cataracts. If you are taking corticosteroids and wish to stop, do not quit suddenly or significantly reduce the amount you are taking. Either of these actions can result in severe withdrawal symptoms. Consult with your doctor before you begin to reduce your drug use.

SUPER ASPIRINS

The quest to develop a drug or drugs that provides all the benefits now offered by NSAIDs but without the harmful and often serious side effects has recently culminated in announcements by several pharmaceutical companies that such products, referred to as super aspirins, are on the horizon. One proposed drug has been named Celebrex (generic, celecoxib) and is being developed and marketed jointly by Searle and Pfizer,

Inc. Another drug is under development by Merck and has been named Vioxx (generic, rofecoxib), and Johnson & Johnson and Glaxo Wellcome each also have a COX-2 drug under development. All these products belong to the same new drug classification called COX-2 inhibitors and are expected to be available on the market by prescription by the middle of 1999 or early in 2000. Celebrex was the first COX-2 inhibitor to receive FDA approval for treatment of arthritis on 1 December 1998.

"Super aspirin" is a term used to describe this new classification of drugs more correctly known as COX-2 inhibitors. COX-2 is an enzyme, cyclooxygenase-2, which is responsible for producing pain and inflammation, characteristics of diseases such as rheumatoid arthritis, osteoarthritis, and fibromyalgia. Super aspirins, such as Vioxx and Celebrex, inhibit the action of COX-2 without affecting the action of COX-1, or cyclooxygenase-1, an enzyme that protects the stomach lining.

What is the difference between NSAIDs (including regular aspirin) and the super aspirins?

The difference between aspirin and other NSAIDs and super aspirins lies in how the two groups of drugs deal with the COX enzymes,

COX-1 and COX-2. COX-1 enzymes are good guys: they help protect the stomach lining against irritants and keep the stomach, kidneys, and other tissues performing smoothly. COX-2 enzymes are the "bad" guys: they cause pain and inflammation. Aspirin and other NSAIDs block the action of both enzymes, thus you get relief from pain and inflammation, but likely pay the price of stomach problems. Super aspirins are formulated so that they stop the action of COX-2 enzymes only; the COX-1 enzymes are free to do their preventive work.

How were super aspirins discovered?

The stage was set for the discovery of COX-2 inhibitors back in 1971 when John Vane, a British researcher and Nobel Prize winner, discovered that aspirin works by blocking the production of prostaglandins, chemicals that cause inflammation, pain, redness, and swelling. To do that, aspirin inhibits the activity of cyclooxygenase. At the time, Vane did not know there was more than one COX enzyme.

In the late 1980s, a researcher named Phillip Needleman, who was then the chairmen of the Pharmacology Department at Washington University in St. Louis, hypothesized that there were two kinds of COX enzymes, COX-1 and COX-2. Needleman further believed that blocking the action of COX-2 would control or prevent inflammation without affecting the action of COX-1. Other scientists conducted studies that confirmed these ideas and isolated COX-2. Beginning in 1991, Needleman and a team of scientists developed a compound which blocked COX-2 but not COX-1. The result was called Celebra (now Celebrex), which was administered to the first test patient in March 1995.

In the meantime, researchers at Merck have also been working on a COX-2 inhibitor, which they named Vioxx. Both Celebrex and Vioxx are the first entrants in the new drug classification of COX-2 inhibitors.

Are the super aspirins more effective than aspirin and NSAIDs?

The COX-2 inhibitors are not more effective, but they are safer and more convenient to use. Super aspirins provide excellent relief of pain and inflammation and improve physical function in people with osteoarthritis and rheumatoid arthritis, and other forms of arthritis. They also relieve the pain associated with dental surgery and menstrual cramps.

In the case of Celebrex, for example, it appeared to work nearly as well as the prescription NSAID naproxen in patients with osteoarthritis and nearly as well as the NSAID diclofenac in patients with rheumatoid arthritis. About 13,000 patients were tested.

Unlike NSAIDs, however, these new drugs are easy on the stomach, so they can be taken in larger doses for a longer time without causing damage to the stomach or kidneys. Scientists report that the serious gastrointestinal side effects associated with NSAIDs do not occur in people who take the COX-2 inhibitors, even at doses ten times the amount used in the clinical studies. Super aspirins also have the advantage of requiring once-daily dosing rather than the two or more needed with NSAIDs.

Some researchers have suggested that COX-2 inhibitors may have the potential to modify the underlying disease, which means use of super aspirins may result in physical improvement in addition to providing symptom relief. For now, this idea is speculation and the subject of additional studies.

Do COX-2 inhibitors have any side effects?

A major advantage of the super aspirins over conventional aspirin and NSAIDs is that the COX-2 inhibitors do not cause the gastrointestinal side effects. However, there is still some risk of ulcers, though small. Researchers for Celebrex performed endoscopic testing (placement of a tube into the stomach to view digestive functioning) on 4,700 individuals to see if the new drug would cause ulcers. They found that between 25 and 40 percent of patients who were taking ibuprofen or naproxen developed mini-ulcers compared with 5 to 10 percent of patients taking Celebrex.

Other adverse effects associated with use of COX-2 inhibitors include diarrhea, edema, insomnia, headache, and upper respiratory infections, which may be caused by a breakdown in the immune system. Investigators for Vioxx, for example, have noted that some elderly patients develop swollen ankles when taking the drug. Overall, however, the elderly tolerate the drug very well. Because the COX-2 inhibitors are new, FDA officials warn that the longer term effects are unknown. Researchers of COX-2 drugs also emphasize that although these drugs are being investigated as to their possible use for cancer, Alzheimer's disease, and other serious conditions, it is much too early to make any claims about their effectiveness.

FIVE

❀

MSM and Arthritis

Perhaps one of the most exciting and important characteristics of MSM is its ability to relieve the pain, stiffness, and inflammation associated with arthritis. This finding may bring relief to millions of people. According to the latest Arthritis Foundation figures, nearly 43 million Americans—16 percent of the population—have some form of arthritis, and the number is increasing. By the year 2020, experts believe nearly 60 million Americans will be afflicted by the disease.

The word *arthritis* usually brings to mind the two most common types of the disease—osteoarthritis and rheumatoid arthritis—but there are many more. In fact, *arthritis* is a general term used to describe more than 100 different diseases that involve the cartilage, joints, muscles, tendons, and ligaments, and occasionally other parts of the body. The literal meaning of the word comes from the Greek words *arth*, meaning "joint," and *itis*, meaning "inflammation." Arthritic diseases are characterized by joint pain, with some of the related conditions mainly affecting the bones (as in osteoporosis) and the muscles (as in fibromyalgia).

Many people believe that arthritis affects only the elderly, yet more than 60 percent of people with arthritis are younger than 65, according to the Arthritis Foundation. Included in this population are the approximately 200,000 children who have some form of arthritis, including about 70,000 who have juvenile rheumatoid arthritis.

Arthritis is usually chronic and often debilitating and is responsible for 3 million physician visits per year. In an attempt to get treatment and relief, Americans spend about $65 billion a year on drugs and related treatments. The Arthritis Foundation reports that arthritis is the main cause of disability in the United States. Despite the prevalence of arthritic diseases, the cause of most of them is not known; nor is there a cure. For now, people with arthritis can best manage their disease with lifestyle modifications and natural remedies, including MSM.

This chapter answers questions about the more common types of arthritis and related conditions, including osteoarthritis, rheumatoid arthritis, gout, lupus, juvenile rheumatoid arthritis, ankylosing spondylitis, tendinitis and bursitis, and fibromyalgia. It also explores the role of diet and nutrition in arthritis, with specific attention to the role of MSM and how it can be used to treat arthritis.

What is osteoarthritis?

Approximately 16 million people in the United States have the degenerative disease known as *osteoarthritis*. Osteoarthritis involves the breakdown of the cartilage in various joints, which usually results in pain and stiffness. It is the most common type of arthritis and most often affects people 50 years of age and older. By age 75, nearly everyone has at least one joint that is affected by osteoarthritis, but not everyone has symptoms. Women generally get the disease earlier than do men.

What are the symptoms of osteoarthritis?

Osteoarthritis is characterized by pain in the joints, caused by the deterioration of the cartilage. The joints most often affected include the base of the thumb, the end joints of the fingers, the joints of the lower back, and the hip and knee. During the early stages of the disease, pain occurs after activity and resolves with rest. As cartilage deterioration progresses, pain occurs even without movement, and many people eventually lose their ability to move the affected joint or limb.

Over time, the muscles surrounding the joints may weaken and shrink if they are not exercised. Therefore even though movement of inflamed joints can be somewhat painful, in the long run it will help strengthen the muscles and support the joint. When knee and hip joints are affected by osteoarthritis, posture, coordination, and gait are often hampered. Some individuals have difficulty walking any distance and require assistance with a cane or walker.

What is rheumatoid arthritis?

Rheumatoid arthritis (RA) is an incurable progressive disease in which the cells of the immune system attack healthy cells in the joint cartilage. This condition, which belongs to a category of diseases known as autoimmune diseases (in which the body attacks itself), can eventually lead to severe joint deformity and greatly limit a person's mobility and quality of life. Rheumatoid arthritis disease affects approximately 1 percent of the world's population and about 2 million Americans. It typically first appears between the ages of 25 and 50, although symptoms can begin at any age. Women are afflicted about two to three times more often than men.

What are the symptoms of rheumatoid arthritis?

Symptoms include inflamed, painful joints and limited range of motion, most often of the joints in the hands and feet, wrists, shoulders, jaw, neck, hips, ankles, and knees. Some people also experience redness over the affected joints and swelling of the eyes and nerves in the arms and legs. Rheumatoid arthritis is often associated with cardiovascular disease, hypertension, pulmonary disease, and infections.

Why is rheumatoid arthritis hard to diagnose?

Overall, rheumatoid arthritis can be difficult to diagnose because it often develops slowly and with subtle symptoms. To help physicians identify this crippling disease, the American Rheumatism Association established specific criteria. Your physician will examine you and ask questions about the following symptoms:

1. Stiffness or inactivity in and around joints in the morning after waking up and for at least one hour before maximum improvement.

2. Swelling or accumulation of fluid in the soft tissues of three or more of the joint areas in the fingers and thumb, as observed by a clinician, as well as the wrist, elbow, knee, and ankle joints.

3. Bilateral swelling of the same joints as mentioned in 2.

4. Swelling of at least one wrist, finger, or thumb joint.

5. Rheumatoid nodules (inflamed bumps or knots that appear over specific areas such as the elbow and wrist).

6. An abnormal level of serum rheumatoid factor (an antibody in the blood that identifies RA from other types of arthritis).

7. Erosion and/or abnormal bony decalcification in or near hand and wrist joints.

To make a diagnosis of rheumatoid arthritis, four or more of the above criteria are required, and criteria 1 through 4 must appear for at least six weeks. If your symptoms fit those listed above, chances are very good, although not definite, that you have rheumatoid arthritis. Although all joints are at risk, those most often affected include the hands, wrists, and feet.

What are some other common types of arthritis?

Like rheumatoid arthritis, *lupus*, also known as systemic lupus erythematosus, is an autoimmune disorder. In people with lupus, the body's cells can attack nearly every bodily organ or system and cause them to become inflamed. This misdirected reaction can be life-threatening, especially when it affects vital organs such as the kidneys, lungs, and heart.

Nearly 240,000 people in the United States have or are strongly suspected of having lupus. This chronic inflammatory disease is characterized by fever, arthritis, fatigue, muscle weakness, and rash. More women than men are affected, and black women have a much higher prevalence than do white women (408 cases per 100,000 vs. 100 per 100,000). (For more on how MSM can help patients who have lupus, see chapter 9.)

Gout is painful inflammation of the joints caused by an excess of uric acid, a chemical naturally produced in the body. Drinking alcohol and eating meat can raise the level of uric acid in the body. Gout pain usually affects one joint at a time, comes on suddenly, and is generally accompanied by redness, swelling, and tenderness. It affects men nearly twice as often as it does women. More than one million Americans have gout.

The joint most often affected is the large one in the big toe. An attack may last several days and can occur after an unusual amount of stress, a serious illness, or an accident.

Fibromyalgia is a debilitating rheumatic disease that afflicts women more often than men. The word *fibromyalgia* means pain in the muscles and the ligaments and tendons that connect them. Symptoms include persistent pain and stiffness in the soft tissues and muscles around the joints rather than arthritis of a joint, and fatigue. Although there is no joint damage or physical deformity associated with fibromyalgia, the constant pain and exhaustion are debilitating and have a serious negative impact on quality of life.

Arthritis affects approximately 200,000 children (from birth to 16 years of age) in the United States. Of these, about 70,000 have *juvenile rheumatoid arthritis*, a disease that can affect both the joints and the internal organs. Symptoms tend to change frequently, with mild pain one day and severe stiffness the next.

Another form of arthritis that often begins in early life is *ankylosing spondylitis*. This disease, which usually first appears among people who are in their late teens or early twenties, affects the spine and peripheral joints. If it is not diagnosed and treated properly, it can cause the spine and rib cage to become rigid, resulting in an inability to turn, bend, or even breathe properly. Ankylosing spondylitis has a genetic cause in more than 90 percent of cases. Researchers have identified a genetic marker for the disease and are in the process of locating others.

Tendinitis and *bursitis*, although often mentioned together, are two different arthritis-like conditions that affect more than 4 million Americans. Often dubbed the "weekend warrior" afflictions, tendinitis and bursitis are rheumatic disorders that are caused by overuse of joints, usually the elbow, ankle, fingers, wrist, and knee. People who are overenthusiastic runners, golfers, and tennis players are some of the individuals who most often get tendinitis or bursitis. In *bursitis*, the small fluid-filled sacs called *bursae* that protect the joints from impact become inflamed when they are under abnormal pressure. *Tendinitis* is the inflammation or irritation of the tendons, the fibrous tissue that connects bones and muscle. When tendons are swollen, they can be very painful to move. Both tendinitis and bursitis are usually temporary conditions but can become chronic if preventive measures are not taken.

Other less common types of arthritis include Lyme disease, psoriatic arthritis, Reiter's syndrome, scleroderma, pseudogout, polymyositis, dermatomyositis, Sjogren's syndrome, temporal arteritis, and Behcet's syndrome.

What are the traditional treatments for arthritis?

Depending on the type and extent of the disease, arthritis is traditionally treated with various medications to control pain, inflammation, and stiffness, and a routine of exercises and/or physical therapy to strengthen the muscles around the joints. The most commonly prescribed medications are nonsteroidal anti-inflammatory drugs (NSAIDs), disease-modifying drugs, and cortisone-type drugs. These are discussed in detail in chapter 4.

Why is arthritis such a widespread problem?

Medical researchers are not certain what causes most types of arthritis, but they have some theories. In the case of the most prevalent form of the disease, osteoarthritis, risk factors seem to be age (risk increases as people age), female sex, obesity, genetic predisposition, and repeated stress or trauma to one or more specific joints. Both genetics and infectious agents are believed to be causes of rheumatoid arthritis. Other significant factors include diet, lifestyle, and environmental influences.

What effect does diet have on arthritis?

An area of great debate is the impact of diet on arthritis. Obesity is a recognized problem for people with arthritis. Many of the joints affected by arthritis are weight-bearing, therefore excess stress on those joints have an obvious detrimental impact. Because diet is one thing people can change themselves if they want to, it is an area many individuals look to for relief of arthritis pain. One problem with this idea is that there are few well-controlled studies of the effect of food and nutrition on arthritis. (The exception is gout, for which there is a clearly defined relationship between intake of uric acid, found in meat, and disease symptoms.)

However, some arthritis patients report that they get positive results when they eliminate certain foods from their diet. It appears that some people are susceptible to specific foods, which may make their pain and swelling worse. One particular fad arthritis diet to avoid is the Alfalfa Diet, in which people are encouraged to consume large amounts of alfalfa. Large amounts of alfalfa can interfere with normal blood cell production.

I've heard about a Nightshade Diet and the Dong Diet. Is there any proof that these work for arthritis?

The Nightshade Diet emerged in the 1960s and was based on the work of a horticulturist at Rutgers University who experienced sore joints after eating vegetables that belong to the nightshade family—potatoes, eggplant, bell peppers, and tomatoes. Although there is no scientific proof that eliminating these foods from your diet will relieve your pain, many people claim that it does. Similarly, the Dong Diet, developed by Collin Dong, M.D., calls for people to eliminate red meat, alcohol, dairy products, fruit, and foods with preservatives and additives. Although there is no scientific evidence to support Dr. Dong's claims, many people do find relief when eliminating meat and dairy from their diet, especially people who have gout.

Is there any truth to the idea that fasting helps relieve arthritis?

Several studies have shown that people with rheumatoid arthritis experience temporary relieve of their joint pain and inflammation when they fast for 7 to 10 days. Fasting is not a practical long-term therapy and unsupervised fasting is dangerous. However, observations of fasting in arthritis patients provides support to the argument that diet affects joint inflammation.

Besides MSM, are there any specific nutritional supplements that may help alleviate arthritis?

Some researchers believe certain nutrients can help some people with arthritis. Among people with rheumatoid arthritis, for example, deficiencies of vitamin D, folic acid, vitamin C, vitamin B_6, iron, selenium, and zinc are common. Similarly, children with juvenile rheumatoid arthritis have low blood levels of zinc, copper, and iron. So far, however, it is not clear whether poor nutrition causes these types of arthritis or whether the deficiencies are the result of the disease itself. A further discussion of diet and arthritis and the possible benefits of nutritional supplements is in chapter 6. A list of nutrients, their RDAs, and their Suggested Therapeutic Dosages is presented in chapter 3, pages 44–45.

What role do heavy metals and environmental toxins play in arthritis?

Over time, the body accumulates toxins from food, such as pesticides, herbicides, food additives, and hormones, as well as poisons from the environment. Dr. Marcellus Walker explains that most people who have joint pain, inflammation, and stiffness experience such problems because the body stores these toxins in the tissues and joints. The longer the poisons stay in the body, the more damage they can cause. MSM has been used to successfully eliminate toxins from the body.

Can a dietary deficiency of MSM be a cause of arthritis?

Researchers around the world have been investigating the relationship between MSM and arthritis. They have found that the concentration of sulfur in the cartilage of people with arthritis is about one-third the level compared to that of normal tissue. This is not a new finding. During the 1930s, researchers reported similar low levels of sulfur in patients with arthritis, and at the time some doctors injected sulfur into the joints of patients with arthritis, with some success.

The recent study also found that the level of cystine, one of the sulfur-containing amino acids, is usually lower in arthritic individuals than in the normal population. Thus a deficiency of sulfur appears to be a characteristic of people with arthritis, although not necessarily a cause. The exact nature of the relationship between sulfur and arthritis is not yet known.

How can MSM help people who have arthritis?

Based on years of research studies by Drs. Jacob and Herschler at Oregon Health Sciences University as well as those of other investigators, many patients with osteoarthritis and rheumatoid arthritis experience excellent relief from pain, inflammation, and stiffness when taking

MSM. Use of MSM compared very favorably with that of conventional medications in its ability to relieve pain. When MSM was compared with ibuprofen (Motrin), for example, MSM provided similar pain relief and anti-inflammatory benefits but without the adverse effects or toxicity associated with use of the drug. Overall, use of MSM has none of the adverse effects associated with conventional medications for arthritis and associated disorders. (These medications are discussed in detail in chapter 4.)

Dozens of clinical reports show that consistent use of MSM reduces inflammation and swelling, which in turn reduces or eliminates the pain and stiffness of osteoarthritis and rheumatoid arthritis. Dr. Walker believes that the people who can reap the most benefit from taking MSM are those who have significant toxicity in their joints and tissues, which the sulfur can help eliminate from the body.

I have arthritis and want to take MSM, but how do I know if I have low levels of MSM in my body?

One of the amazing things about the human body is that every person has his or her own unique chemical makeup. Within limits, levels and amounts of each of the proteins, vitamins, minerals, enzymes, hormones, and other substances fluctuate and are affected by diet, stress, heredity, and environmental influences. If you want to give your body what it really needs to operate at its best, it makes sense to make sure it needs what you want to give it. According to Hunter Yost, M.D., a nutritional orthomolecular physician practicing in Tucson, Arizona, it is wise to determine what your body may be lacking before you begin to take supplements. This not only helps ensure you will get the relief you need but also avoids wasting time, energy, and money pursuing remedies your body does not require.

One way to make that determination is to have the Standard Detoxification Profile, a blood and urine analysis performed by Great Smokies Diagnostic Laboratory in North Carolina. This test identifies the degree of toxin exposure and the level of nutrients in the body. Dr. Yost also recommends undergoing a nutritional blood chemistry analysis. Together these tests will identify your body's specific nutritional needs and allow you and your physician to choose the most beneficial course of action for you.

Dr. Marcellus Walker agrees that the Standard Detoxification Profile is a good first step to determine the need for MSM. He also uses a technique called applied kinesiology to perform a muscle test which involves the use of light finger pressure on specific points on the body to identify nutritional deficiencies. Dr. Walker believes most people are deficient in sulfur and can benefit from MSM, although the need should be established before arbitrarily taking supplements.

How much MSM should I take to relieve my arthritis?

No definitive therapeutic guidelines for MSM have been established for treating the pain associated with arthritis. However, you may want to follow the advice of Dr. Jacob, who reports that 2,000 to 5,000 mg per day, divided into 2 to 4 equal doses, is a good therapeutic regimen for the first 2 to 4 weeks of treatment. Most people who begin with this course of treatment notice results within 2 to 21 days. Then, as the pain subsides, you can switch to a maintenance dose of 250 to 750 mg per day. If you experience a flare-up of pain or other symptoms, increase the dosage until symptoms are under control.

This is only a suggested dosing schedule. The best dosage for you will depend on the severity of your disease, the amount of MSM already in your system, and the cause of your symptoms. If you want to take a high dosage of MSM, it is best to consult with your health-care practitioner.

I want to try MSM for osteoarthritis. What kind of results are people getting with MSM for this kind of arthritis?

Relief of arthritis symptoms seems to be the number one reason people use MSM. Generally the response is very positive. Many people report they have used MSM daily for two years and longer with continuous good response and no side effects. MSM has enabled many people to completely eliminate their need for analgesics or NSAIDs, which in turn rids them of worrying about or experiencing the accumulative effects of those drugs.

How long will I need to take MSM for arthritis pain?

MSM is not a silver bullet: a single dose will not bring instant relief from pain, stiffness, and swelling. However, because MSM is nontoxic when taken as directed, many experts believe you can take moderate amounts (250 to 2,000 mg per day) indefinitely without fear of adverse effects and toxicity. If you want to take MSM simply as a dietary supplement to help maintain your body's sulfur levels, 250 to 500 mg per day is usually sufficient. If you want to treat specific symptoms or have a severe condition, researchers have found that doses of 2,000 to 5,000 mg per day have been taken for up to 6 months without adverse effects. To provide the most effective therapeutic benefit, MSM must be taken every day.

I've read that some people take vitamin C along with MSM for arthritis. What type of benefit can I expect by taking these two supplements together?

Some patients with arthritis report increased relief when they combine MSM and vitamin C. Taking these two supplements together may be beneficial because MSM and vitamin C work together to build new cells. Vitamin C needs to be taken daily because it is water soluble (and so cannot be stored in the body) and because the body constantly draws upon its supply of vitamin C to manufacture new cells, thus rapidly depleting the supply. Vitamin C also is a powerful antioxidant—a substance that fights free radicals in the body. Free radicals are highly charged molecules that can cause cell damage and a breakdown of the immune system. Sufficient vitamin C is needed to work along with sulfur to prevent cell damage and an opportunity for infection to take hold.

When you take more than 1,000 mg of vitamin C per day, it helps your body increase its natural production of the anti-inflammatory substance cortisone and enhances the immune system. A healthy immune system is always important, but especially if you have rheumatoid arthritis or any other autoimmune disease. For maximum benefit, take equal amounts of vitamin C and MSM. If you take 2,000 mg of MSM per day, for example, take 1,000 mg each of MSM and vitamin C in the morning and the same dose at night.

Are there other natural supplements I can take along with MSM to treat arthritis?

All studies with MSM have shown that it is completely compatible with natural remedies as well as food and medication. A detailed discussion of some of the natural supplements that complement treatment with MSM can be found in chapter 6.

One herbal remedy that complements the pain relieving and anti-inflammatory actions of MSM very well is ginger. Zinaxin® and other ginger extracts are discussed in detail in chapter 7.

One note of caution comes from Dr. Herschler. He found that DMSO, if taken along with MSM, rapidly eliminates MSM from the body via the kidneys. Therefore anyone who takes both supplements will not derive any benefit from MSM.

SIX

Using MSM With Other Natural Remedies for Arthritis

The use of herbs, nutrients, and other natural supplements as treatment for arthritis and other medical problems is growing among complementary medicine practitioners as well as those who practice more conventional medicine. But perhaps the group most interested in these alternative remedies are people like you, the patients themselves. You, along with your health-care providers, are discovering the benefits and pitfalls of these treatment options and how they complement the healing actions of MSM.

One reason for this shift in health care is that the use of drugs to treat arthritis is problematic. One reason is that relief is temporary, a "Band-Aid" solution. In order to keep getting relief, you need to keep taking the drugs, often in increasing amounts to get the same level of resolution. Adverse effects, like those caused by aspirin and NSAIDs, then become medical problems you need to resolve. What you then have created is a cycle of taking drugs to resolve one problem, only to have new symptoms arise, which you then treat with more drugs. The result is a no-win situation that affects both your physical and your emotional health.

Another downside of drugs is that although analgesics and anti-inflammatory medications kill pain and reduce swelling, they do not change the cause of these symptoms, so they return, again and again, as the joints continue to be damaged.

In this chapter, you can learn about the most effective natural supplements you can take along with MSM for treatment of arthritis. This chapter also looks at the use of exercise as a form of arthritis therapy and the part stress plays in arthritis symptoms.

NATURAL REMEDIES THAT COMPLEMENT MSM FOR ARTHRITIS

The body naturally produces several sulfur-containing compounds that play vital roles in maintaining health. Some of these compounds also have significant healing powers when taken as a supplement. The potential for all of these substances to perform their best may be enhanced when you take them along with MSM to contribute sulfur. Several of the more common sulfur-containing agents are discussed below, as well as a few other natural supplements that some physicians and patients are using along with MSM.

Glucosamine sulfate has received a lot of attention as a treatment for osteoarthritis. What is glucosamine?

Glucosamine sulfate is a sulfur-containing compound that occurs naturally in all body tissues. One of its major functions is to help cushion the joints and surrounding tissues, which makes it a vital factor in the relief of the symptoms of osteoarthritis. It also gives cartilage its structure, strength, and resiliency.

Should I take glucosamine for osteoarthritis?

The body's ability to support healthy cell growth and repair decreases as people age. The addition of glucosamine to the diet, especially as a supplement, helps the body replace old and worn-out cells and tissues. This in turn helps relieve the pain, inflammation, and limited mobility associated with osteoarthritis.

Unlike conventional medications, which mask symptoms and can even stimulate the disease process, glucosamine sulfate can improve symptoms and in some cases eliminate them and repair damaged joints. Glucosamine is sometimes used in combination with MSM and another sulfur-containing agent called chondroitin sulfate, which also occurs naturally in the body.

Does chondroitin sulfate do the same thing as glucosamine for arthritis?

Unlike glucosamine, which repairs cells, chondroitin sulfate prevents the destructive action of the enzymes that break down old cartilage. Both glucosamine and chondroitin have been used by Europeans to treat osteoarthritis since 1980. Before the mid 1990s in the United States, chondroitin and glucosamine were used primarily to treat arthritis in dogs and horses. Since then these two supplements have exploded into the consumer market and now are available in more than 100 versions, both singly and as a combined supplement (see appendix B). According to Jason Theodosakis, M.D., author of *The Arthritis Cure*, glucosamine and chondroitin can "slow, halt, or prevent the degeneration of cartilage."

How do I take glucosamine and chondroitin?

Based on the results of studies and the recommendations of physicians who both prescribe and use these supplements themselves, including Dr. Theodosakis, the suggested daily intake for individuals who are between 120 and 200 pounds is 1,500 mg for glucosamine and 1,200 mg for chondroitin. Individuals who weigh less than 120 pounds should take 1,000 mg glucosamine plus 800 mg chondroitin. The dosage for people who weigh more than 200 pounds is 2,000 mg glucosamine plus 1,600 mg chondroitin.

Both supplements can be taken along with MSM. Once you experience symptom relief, gradually decrease the amount of the supplements until you reach a point where your symptoms are well managed.

Some doctors, like James McKoy, M.D., a rheumatologist at Kaiser Permanente of Hawaii, in Honolulu, find that glucosamine alone is sufficient for symptom relief. Dr. McKoy recommends 500 mg of glucosamine taken three times a day, which he says provides the same amount of pain relief as does 1,200 mg of ibuprofen. The problem with chondroitin, he says, is that many of the studies used an injectable form of the supplement while consumers largely have access to the pill form, which is not well absorbed by the body.

How long will it take to see results when I take glucosamine and chondroitin?

Glucosamine, chondroitin, and MSM can be taken along with NSAIDs, but the drugs should be stopped after six to eight weeks to see whether the natural supplements have taken effect. Not everyone experiences relief. If you have not experienced satisfactory pain relief after several months of taking the supplements, you probably will not benefit from them. Dr. McKoy says most patients who are going to get relief will begin to experience noticeable results within six to eight weeks. If you have advanced arthritis and much cartilage loss, the supplements probably will not help you.

Are there any precautions associated with the use of glucosamine and chondroitin?

These supplements should not be taken if you are pregnant or could get pregnant. If you have diabetes and want to take glucosamine, check your blood sugar levels often. Although no problems have been noted in humans, glucosamine has caused an increase in blood sugar in some animals.

David Hungerford, M.D., a professor of orthopedic surgery and chief of arthritis surgery at Johns Hopkins University School of Medicine in Baltimore, notes that glucosamine is indicated for osteoarthritis but not for rheumatoid arthritis or gout. He urges people with undiagnosed joint pain to see a doctor rather than self-treat with what may prove to be an inappropriate and ineffective remedy.

The consensus among physicians is that glucosamine and chondroitin supplements appear to be safe and might reduce pain in 30 to 50 percent of patients with osteoarthritis. They warn, however, that because these substances are marketed as food supplements, they are not regulated by the Food and Drug Administration. Consumers are urged to buy only high-quality products from reputable manufacturers.

I read an article that recommended taking niacinamide with glucosamine and chondroitin. What are the benefits of this combination for arthritis?

Some health-care practitioners recommend niacinamide (vitamin B_3; do not confuse it with niacin) for people who have severe osteoarthritis. According to some patients, the niacinamide seems to make the gluosamine and chondroitin more effective. The suggested dose of niacinamide is 250 mg three times daily. Niacinamide has proved to be safe in long-term studies and to not cause toxic effects.

I've heard that glutathione can help arthritis. What is glutathione?

Nearly all life forms on Earth have some of the sulfur-containing amino acid glutathione. This compound is composed of three amino acids: glycine, glutamic acid, and the sulfur-bearing amino acid cysteine. Glutathione is manufactured by the body and is most concentrated in the liver, kidneys, spleen, and pancreas. It is also available as a synthetic supplement. Collectively the three elements in glutathione perform vital functions, as does each of them individually.

Why is glutathione important in arthritis?

Like MSM, one of glutathione's primary tasks is to remove waste from the body, including the toxins that accumulate in the joints and synovial fluid. Glutathione molecules attach to toxins in the liver and allow the liver to excrete the poisons without any damage occurring to this vital organ. It also has a reputation as a "smart nutrient" because it protects against a process called "cross-linking" of proteins, which can cause brain cell function to decline.

Individually, each of the three amino acids in glutathione has specific duties. Cysteine helps protect against environmental toxins and prevents aging and cancer. Glutamic acid assists in the metabolism of fats and sugars and produces a substance called GABA, which has a calming effect on the brain and helps reduce cravings for alcohol and sugar. Glycine stimulates production of glutathione and aids in the detoxification process.

Low levels of glutathione are associated with high levels of cholesterol, higher body weight, and various eye diseases. Because glutathione helps fight cancer, stabilize blood sugar, and repair cells, insufficient levels can be especially stressful and damaging to the body. Sufficient intake of MSM is necessary to maintain healthy levels of glutathione.

Why should I take a glutathione supplement?

The amount of glutathione in the body declines as people age. You can include more foods in your diet that contain the sulfur amino acids, or you can take a cysteine supplement, which helps build glutathione (see chapter 2). Supplementation is the preferred approach.

A friend told me that I should be taking essential fatty acids for my arthritis. What are essential fatty acids?

Essential fatty acids are fats the body needs to perform its functions but cannot manufacture itself. Therefore they must be obtained through diet. Their primary task is to strengthen cell membranes and participate in the growth of muscle and nerve tissue.

What effect do essential fatty acids have on arthritis?

Several essential fatty acids have specific therapeutic abilities, but the ones you need to pay attention to are the omega-3s (eicosapentaenoic acid and docosahexanoic acid). Omega-3 fatty acids are anti-inflammatories and also help prevent heart disease. Arnold Fox, M.D., who uses MSM for his arthritis patients, also recommends essential fatty acids, which he calls "very, very important. They do what the prescription medications can do." What essential fatty acids do is suppress the action of the substances that cause inflammation, namely, "bad" prostaglandins and leukotrienes, and help ensure the production of the "good" prostaglandins. On a physical level, you can expect improvement in morning stiffness when you take omega-3 supplements.

Another essential fatty acid you may hear about is omega-6. These fatty acids are found in vegetable oils (e.g., sunflower, soy, sesame, and safflower) and produce inflammatory chemicals in the body. It is best to avoid foods that contain these oils.

How can I add omega-3 fatty acids to my diet?

Omega-3 fatty acids are found in hemp seed oil and in fish oils, particularly cold-water fish such as salmon, mackerel, sardines, and herring. Dr. Theodosakis, author of *The Arthritis Cure*, recommends eating fish two to five times a week, or taking 1 to 2 teaspoons of fish oil daily. (Note: Fish oil can be toxic if taken in large amounts. Do not exceed the recommended dosage.) Alternatives to these suggestions include taking 200 to 300 mg evening primrose oil, black currant oil, or borage seed oil daily. *In rare cases, these oils may trigger inflammation.*

Should I take vitamin supplements for my arthritis?

Some scientific studies show that people with arthritis can benefit from certain nutrients. Although it is always best to get your nutrients from nature—fruits, vegetables, grains, legumes, seeds, and nuts—supplements are often necessary for several reasons. You may want to eat healthy foods, and hopefully you do, at least most of the time. But sometimes you may not have the time or means to make sure you eat healthy meals. And many factors can have a negative impact on how your body absorbs and uses nutrients. Chronic stress, environmental pollutants, lack of sleep, and use of tobacco, alcohol, or drugs can hinder how the body utilizes nutrients. A chronic disease such as arthritis also can affect how your body absorbs and uses nutrients, or you may be taking a medication that interferes with nutrient absorption. In particular, arthritis can deplete the body's supply of vitamins A, B_6, C, and E, and the nutrients selenium, pantothenic acid, and copper.

To find out if you are deficient in any nutrient or if taking a particular supplement may help you, it is best to undergo a nutritional analysis, which your doctor can arrange for you (see chapter 5, "How do I know if I have low levels of MSM in my body?").

Are there any specific vitamins that can help relieve or prevent arthritis?

Some nutrients and supplements can be beneficial for certain forms of arthritis. Although they do not work for all people who have arthritis, many physicians suggest them for their patients because in some cases they turn out to be an effective, low-cost, and safe alternative to NSAIDs or at least allow patients to reduce their drug dosage.

Physicians on the advisory board of the Arthritis Foundation, for example, have made recommendations based on studies of the relationship between nutrition and arthritis. Essential fatty acids, discussed above, are one recommended nutrient for people with rheumatoid arthritis. Two other nutrients for this group of patients as well as those with lupus are calcium and vitamin D, especially for those who are taking glucocorticoid drugs, such as prednisone, which cause bone loss. If your skin is not exposed to at least 15 minutes of sunlight a day, you should probably take a vitamin D supplement combined with your calcium supplement. Adults need 400 IU vitamin D and 800 to 1,500 mg calcium per day. Vitamin D is also important in people with osteoarthritis. Research has shown that the risk of osteoarthritis progression is three times greater in people who have a low level of vitamin D intake.

Studies of the patients associated with the famous Framingham Heart study have shown that higher intake of the antioxidants vitamin C, vitamin E, and beta-carotene can help reduce the risk of progression of osteoarthritis. Supplementation with folic acid (up to 800 mcg daily) may be helpful for people with rheumatoid arthritis who take methotrexate, as this drug depletes the body of folic acid and can lead to side effects such as diarrhea and nausea.

Which foods are the best sources of these recommended nutrients?

Calcium is usually synonymous with dairy foods; however, milk and other dairy products are best avoided or consumed in small amounts because of their high fat and cholesterol content, the presence of additives, and the fact that many people are sensitive to milk items. Excellent alternatives are calcium-enriched orange juice, broccoli, bok choy, tofu, and spinach and other leafy green vegetables.

Good sources of vitamin C include citrus fruits, all berries, broccoli, kale, potatoes, spinach, brussels sprouts, and peppers. Folic acid is found in abundance in barley, beans, brewer's yeast, endive, most fruits, leafy green vegetables, lentils, oranges, peas, brown rice, soybeans, sprouts, and wheat germ. Vitamin E is found in almonds, oils (corn, cottonseed, safflower, peanut, wheat germ, sunflower), walnuts, wheat germ, whole-grain flour, and filberts. Sources of beta-carotene include apricots, broccoli, cantaloupe, carrots, kale, pumpkin, spinach, squash, and sweet potatoes.

Is there any truth to reports that zinc or copper can help people with rheumatoid arthritis?

Compared with the normal population, people with rheumatoid arthritis have a lower average blood zinc level. Unfortunately, little research has been done to examine this connection. One study involved 24 patients with rheumatoid arthritis who were given zinc pills for 12 days. These patients did experience improvement in their disease, yet such a short trial is not comprehensive enough to be scientifically useful.

The role of copper in rheumatoid arthritis has been studied since the mid twentieth century. Since 1940, more than 1,000 people with rheumatoid arthritis have received copper pills in scientific studies, and the range of improvement has been from 30 to 90 percent. Copper supplements are associated with frequent side effects, including a change in sense of taste and smell, nausea, vomiting, loss of appetite, abnormal blood clots, increased joint pain, chills, and kidney abnormalities. Although copper can be absorbed through the skin, the amount that enters the body through wearing copper bracelets is extremely small. Given the magnitude of side effects and the lack of solid clinical evidence, it is doubtful copper will become a useful treatment for arthritis.

Are there any other natural substances I can take along with MSM to alleviate arthritis pain and inflammation?

A few studies show that herbs such as burdock root and the natural enzyme bromelain, when used in combination with vitamin C and bioflavonoids such as rutin, can be equally or more effective than aspirin and other NSAIDs for reducing pain and inflammation.

Burdock is an excellent blood purifier and works rapidly to reduce the pain and inflammation of rheumatoid arthritis, osteoarthritis, and gout. Burdock is available in capsules, as a powder, or as a dried herb. The suggested dosage is one capsule twice daily, or ½ teaspoon twice daily in water; or you can prepare a tea using one ounce of herb in 12 ounces of boiling water. Drink 3 ounces three to four times a day. Occasionally, burdock may cause slight stomach discomfort, but only if taken in large doses.

Bromelain is a naturally occuring enzyme, found in pineapple, which digests protein. Taken as a supplement, it helps reduce inflammation and stimulates blood circulation. To treat inflammation, take 250 to 500 mg between meals. If you need it as a digestive aid, take the same dose after meals. There are no side effects associated with bromelain.

An effective topical botanical remedy is red pepper, sometimes referred to as capsicum. Red pepper contains painkillers known as salicylates, which are similar to the chemicals found in aspirin; and capsaicin, a compound that promotes the body's release of natural painkillers called endorphins. When applied to painful areas, capsaicin creams are effective pain relievers, especially for people with arthritis. Look for creams that contain 0.025 percent capsaicin (e.g., Capzasin-P, Zostrix). Because some people are sensitive to red pepper, test the cream on a small area of your skin before you apply it to a larger area.

I've heard that ginger is an effective pain reliever and anti-inflammatory. Should I take ginger along with MSM?

The use of ginger extracts to treat arthritis symptoms has risen dramatically because it is a safe, natural approach that has produced some dramatic results. For that reason, an entire chapter is devoted to it; see chapter 7.

NATURAL REMEDIES, CONVENTIONAL DOCTORS, AND YOU

My doctor prescribes painkillers and NSAIDs for arthritis, but I don't like the fact that they are potentially dangerous. I want to try something different. Should I change doctors?

Many physicians still prescribe the NSAIDs for arthritis pain, inflammation, and loss of mobility, but are doing so with increasing caution. Says Arnold Fox, M.D., of Beverly Hills, California and author of many books, including *Immune for Life* and *The Healthy Prostate*, "I could prescribe NSAIDs and sometimes do, for less than a week." He then turns to natural methods, including essential fatty acids, MSM, glucosamine, and chondroitin sulfate. Some physicians gradually wean their patients off drugs and onto natural remedies alone, while others use a combination of conventional and natural approaches.

Talk with your doctor about changing your treatment plan. Ask whether he or she has used some of the complementary remedies. Don't be surprised, however, if your doctor isn't receptive to the idea of using natural remedies. Many doctors are not very familiar with alternatives such as MSM and glucosamine.

What should I do if my doctor isn't familiar with natural remedies or refuses to let me try something different?

That's when you must take your health care into your own hands. Gather all the information you can about the alternative choices available to you. Sources of information include health organizations, journal and magazine articles, books, the Internet, health professionals who prescribe the remedies in their practices, and people who have used such treatments. Find health-care providers in your area who are knowledgeable about these remedies. Talk to people who have gone to these practitioners and about the care they received.

I know where to begin. How do I find a qualified alternative medicine practitioner?

There are organizations for nearly every alternative medicine specialty, and these organizations typically provide a practitioner referral service. A list of sources to help you get started is provided in appendix A. Many cities now also have holistic or natural health clinics, which usually employ a diversified staff of natural health practitioners.

Besides taking natural supplements, what other steps can I take if I want to reduce or eliminate my use of conventional drugs for arthritis?

In addition to MSM and other natural remedies, there are lifestyle modifications you can make to help you better manage arthritis without the need for toxic drugs. Use of heat and cold in the form of hydrotherapy or compresses applied to the affected areas is an effective way to relieve pain and to increase circulation. Ask your doctor or physical therapist for tips on using hydrotherapy.

Attention to your diet is also essential not only for arthritis, but for overall health. Although all the facts are in concerning a connection tween consuming certain foods and arthritis, it appears that at least some people get significant relief from arthritis symptoms by modifying their eating habits (see chapter 5). One connection that has been established is that between MSM and gout.

Appropriate exercises designed to restore range of motion in your joints and increase muscle strength can help stop disease progression. Ask your rheumatologist to recommend a physical therapist, occupational therapist, or other rehabilitative therapist with whom you can develop an exercise program that suits your particular needs. Such a program will include a combination of aerobic training and weight training, with special attention to maintaining the integrity of your affected joints and limbs and preventing deterioration in others.

Finally, stress management can alleviate painful joints. Simple techniques you can teach yourself and do at home, such as meditation, visualization, and self-talk, have been proved to provide relief for people suffering with pain.

Exercising is the last thing I feel like doing. It hurts too much. Won't it make the arthritis even worse?

If the thought of exercising turns you off, consider this: not all the pain you feel is directly caused by the arthritis itself. You probably noticed that as your pain increased, your level of activity decreased. When you stop moving your muscles, they lose their tone, strength, and flexibility. The range of motion in your joints becomes limited, and the deconditioned muscles become tense and cause you pain.

When you begin to exercise these muscles again, you will feel pain and discomfort in the beginning. However, when done carefully and gradually over time, a regular program of exercise can reduce your pain while increasing your mobility, flexibility, and strength. It's important to develop your exercise program with a therapist or your physician to avoid injury or any further damage to the joints.

What are the best kinds of exercise for people who have arthritis?

Both aerobic and strengthening exercises, done in moderation and according to ability, are recommended for people with arthritis. Aerobic exercise is any activity that increases your heart rate and keeps it elevated for 20 consecutive minutes. Walking, jogging, bicycling, rowing, cross-country skiing, swimming, stair climbing, and aerobics classes are some examples. If you experience significant joint pain, swimming and water aerobics can give you a good workout without the burden of weight on your joints.

Exercises that build strength are important because they promote healthy bones and help maintain the health of the joints. Weight lifting using weight machines or free weights is good for improving strength. For improved flexibility, yoga and stretching exercises are recommended.

What are the benefits of exercise for people with arthritis?

Exercise helps keep the joints healthy because it promotes the flow of synovial fluid to cartilage.

It is believed synovial fluid slows the progression of osteoarthritis. Exercise also strengthens the muscles, tendons, bones, and ligaments; improves circulation, sexual function, and balance; promotes relaxation; increases resistance to disease; and improves range of motion and flexibility.

Does stress play any role in arthritis?

Researchers know that emotions such as fear, anger, and despair can increase how one perceives pain as well as the actual level of pain, and arthritis pain is no different. For many people who experience chronic pain, there is a two-way street that occurs: the chronic pain causes constant stress on both the body and mind and can lead to depression; and the emotional stress they feel about having their disease causes muscle tension, which in turn causes pain.

Stress can appear in many forms, especially for people who have chronic pain. Frustration over not being able to function as well as they did before arthritis struck is stressful; so is the toll medications take on the body. There is also the stress of worrying about how much worse the pain may get, whether one is a burden to loved ones, or whether arthritis will prevent one from enjoying a vacation or other special events.

What can I do to reduce the pain and stress without using drugs?

The good news is that you have the power to control your pain. Countless studies in the area of mind-body medicine show that people have the ability to relieve symptoms such as pain and anxiety by using their minds. When you take some control over your pain, you break the cycle into which many people with arthritis fall: pain prevents them from being active and interested in life, which makes them depressed, which leads them to want to do even less, which contributes even more to their pain. Some of the techniques you can use to distract your mind from pain are meditation, biofeedback, self-hypnosis, visualization, and self-talk. For information on these and other ways to manage stress and pain, see appendix A and the list of sources and suggested readings at the back of this book.

❈
SEVEN
❈

The Power of Zinaxin and Other Ginger Extracts

Thousands of years ago, spices such as ginger, cumin, fenugreek, nutmeg, tamarind, aniseed, and black pepper were highly sought after, not only for their flavor but for their power to heal. Spices, like many herbs, were the medicines of our ancestors. Now they have come full circle to join the medicines of today.

The scientific and medical communities have been exploring the plant world and analyzing many herbs and spices and their medicinal powers. One of the spices that caught their eye is ginger, which has been used for millennia for a variety of medical conditions and symptoms. After years of countless clinical trials and reports, several natural ginger extracts are now available on the market and are being sold for several purposes, one of which is to relieve the pain and inflammation associated with arthritis and rheumatic disorders. These ginger products are now often used in conjunction with MSM and other natural remedies for pain and inflammation disorders.

This chapter answers some of the questions about ginger extracts and how you can use them along with MSM to treat arthritis. In particular it explores the development of a new ginger extract called Zinaxin and how it works for arthritis and other medical conditions.

THE STORY OF GINGER

What is ginger, a spice or an herb?

Ginger is not one plant but several species of plants that belong to the Zingiberaceae family and which share very similar characteristics. To identify whether ginger is a spice or an herb, you need a definition of each. *Spices* are the aromatic roots, seeds, rhizomes, or barks of a plant used to flavor food. They are derived from plants that typically grow in hot climates. *Herbs* may also have aromatic components and/or be used as flavorings. They differ, however, in that they consist mainly of leaves and grow primarily in temperate climates. These definitions place ginger squarely in the spice category, because it is grown in hot areas of the world, and the root (or more correctly, the rhizome) is the part used.

What is a rhizome?

When people refer to ginger "root," what they actually mean is the rhizome, or underground stem. The ginger rhizome is a fleshy, bulbous object that looks somewhat like a hand with stubby fingers and a corklike skin that is creamy brown or buff. The roots project out from the rhizome, but these are usually scraped off by the time ginger reaches the market. Ginger can be purchased fresh or dried.

What makes ginger a popular remedy for arthritis?

Like many herbs and spices, ginger's history goes back 5,000 years ago to ancient China, where the Chinese had already discovered the value of the spice to relieve the stiffness and pain associated with arthritic conditions. According to Chinese medicine, which classifies herbs and spices as being warming or cooling substances, ginger is a warming remedy. As such, one of its uses is to treat conditions believed to be caused by the entry of cold and dampness into the body, such as arthritis and rheumatic disorders.

Ginger also was, and still is, a key ingredient

in the world's oldest written health care system. Ayurveda, the "Science of Life," incorporates ginger into most of its tonic formulas because it stimulates function of the body's systems.

The word that ginger was effective in the treatment of pain and inflammation associated with arthritis and similar conditions spread throughout the ages and around the world. It was a highly sought-after spice among the ancient Romans and Egyptians, who used it both in cooking and as a medicinal herb. The ancient Greeks used it to warm the body and to cure digestive problems. In medieval England, it was used to treat the plague.

With such a long and consistent history, it seemed natural for modern-day investigators to analyze ginger for its medicinal powers. And that's what they did.

What have researchers learned about ginger that makes it medically useful?

According to work compiled by James A. Duke, Ph.D., a prominent expert on medical plants and a member of the U.S. Department of Agriculture, ginger consists of many compounds, several of which are the keys to its effectiveness in the fight against arthritis pain. These key ingredients, gingerol and shogaol, have pain-killing and fever-lowering capabilities, and gingerol has the added ability to calm and soothe the stomach. Another ingredient, borneol, also has anti-inflammatory qualities.

Two other ingredients in ginger that are used in the production of the gingerols are gingerdiones and dehydroginerdiones. These elements inhibit the manufacture of substances produced in the body which are responsible for inflammation. Other compounds present in ginger in small quantities but which are known to have painkilling abilities include capsaicin and curcumin (which also has anti-inflammatory properties).

How does ginger work to relieve the symptoms of arthritis?

The two agents in the body that promote pain and inflammation in arthritis are prostaglandins and leukotrienes. The gingerols prevent the body from manufacturing substances known as cyclooxygenase and lipo-oxygenase, which in turn inhibits the production of prostaglandins and leukotrienes. This is how ginger reduces and eliminates joint pain and swelling in arthritis patients.

Why is an herbal product like ginger effective in relieving arthritis symptoms?

Nature packages all the components of a spice or herb into one holistic unit in which all the elements work together, synergistically, to bring about healing. This is one of the things that is special about herbal medicine. Herbal remedies do not simply eliminate symptoms; they actually work at a deeper level and help the body heal itself. And they usually heal without causing any adverse effects like those associated with conventional medicine.

The ginger rhizome, like all plants, contains many different substances, some of which scientists have yet even to discover. The actions of some of these components, such as gingerols, are known by scientists; others are still a mystery. That does not mean, however, that they are not somehow necessary in the total healing picture. That's why although it is important for researchers to identify individual elements in a plant and what each element is capable of doing, it is also essential to ingest the entire essence of the plant, to get the total power of the plant.

Zinaxin

I've heard there's a ginger extract product on the market that is the result of a new extrac-

tion method. What is this new extract?

The product is called Zinaxin HMP-33 (known as Zinax in some parts of the world). Zinaxin HMP-33 is a patented standardized natural extract of ginger rhizome (*Zingiber officinale Roscoe*). Zinaxin HMP-33 was developed by a Danish scientist, Morten Weidner, and is marketed as a medically and scientifically proved treatment for arthritis and rheumatism.

If I take Zinaxin HMP-33, how fast can I expect to get relief?

Zinaxin HMP-33 reportedly provides relief from arthritic and rheumatic pain within 3 to 28 days and does so without any of the gastrointestinal side effects associated with use of NSAIDs.

How is Zinaxin HMP-33 different from other ginger extracts on the market?

Zinaxin HMP-33 reportedly consists of specially chosen ginger that has been derived using a patented extracted procedure. This procedure guarantees the preservation and uniform quality of the active ingredients in the ginger in their natural and stable state. The standardization of Zinaxin also ensures the integrity of the active ingredients within each capsule and from batch to batch, and eliminates the possibility of causing gastrointestinal problems.

According to the manufacturer, Eurovita A/S Denmark, Zinaxin is absorbed faster, reaches a greater blood level, and maintains that level for a longer time than do other ginger extracts. Zinaxin HMP-33 is able to do this, says Arne Skjold Iversen, M.D., medical director of Eurovita, because their researchers discovered the importance of what they call the "carrier," a molecule that binds to the active substance in ginger and which is necessary for effective absorption of the active ingredients.

There are other ginger extract products on the market that have also been produced using individualized extraction methods. You may want to explore the merits of several extracts before making a decision as to which extract to purchase. See appendix B for a list of other ginger extract products and manufacturers.

What kind of studies have been done with Zinaxin?

Danish scientists have done many clinical trials and three larger studies in osteoarthritis with Zinaxin HMP-33. One study, conducted by Dr. Henning Bliddal, head of rheumatology at the Copenhagen Municipal Hospital, involved 56 people with osteoarthritis of the hip and knee. Dr. Bliddal compared the effectiveness of Zinaxin with that of ibuprofen (an NSAID) and placebo. He reported that "Zinax is the first herbal drug which has been shown to have a measurable effect in a controlled study of osteoarthritis." No side effects were observed.

Another study, this one by Dr. M. Norgaard in Copenhagen, was conducted over a three-month period and involved 28 patients who had had polyarthritis for 7 to 35 years. Significant improvement in stiffness and/or pain was reported by 25 of the 28 patients, and again no side effects were reported.

The latest study done on Zinaxin HMP-33, conducted in the United States as a multicenter, placebo-controlled project, indicated mixed results. Some of the 86 patients who completed the study experienced marginally significant improvement when taking the ginger extract and significant improvement on several of the secondary study parameters, such as how much pain they felt when standing. Improvement was not significant, however, on the primary parameter, even though the dose was similar to that used in previous studies. These findings prompted the researchers to enhance the potency of the extract.

How was Zinaxin HMP-33 improved?

To enhance the effectiveness of Zinaxin, the investigators studied other members of the Zingiberaceae family. They found that *Alpinia galanga L* works synergistically with *Zingiber officinale R* in animal studies. The result of their work is Zinaxin HMP-33/3, which contains both species of ginger. The new formulation is three to five times stronger than its predecessor in reducing swelling in the paws of rats.

What are some of the other uses for Zinaxin?

A series of published clinical studies have verified that ginger extract is effective in reducing symptoms of seasickness and postoperative nausea, and in eliminating morning sickness. New research on the species *Alpinia galanga L* in particular shows that it has certain elements which possess antitumor and antifungal properties. Further studies are needed to determine whether these qualities will be useful in fighting cancer and fungal infections.

What is the recommended dosage of Zinaxin?

The standard dosage suggested for people with osteoarthritis, rheumatoid arthritis, fibromyalgia, and other arthritis-related conditions is two capsules per day, taken with liquid, one in the morning and the other in the evening, for a period of one month. After the first month, take one to two capsules per day as needed. Each of the new Zinaxin HMP-33/3 capsules contains 255 mg of HMP-33/3, which corresponds to 3,000 mg *Zingiber officinale R* (rhizome) and 3,000 mg *Alpinia galanga L* (rhizome).

Buying and Using Ginger Extracts

I want to use fresh ginger. How do I prepare it?

You can purchase fresh ginger rhizome from Oriental grocery stores, herb stores, farmers' markets, or from some supermarkets. The rhizome can be grated using a cheese grater. One level teaspoon of grated fresh ginger equals about 4 grams or a 100mg tablet of concentrated ginger. One-quarter teaspoon of dried ginger equals 1 gram, or a 100mg tablet of concentrated ginger.

A report in *Medical Hypothesis* (29: 25–28, 1989) showed that people with rheumatoid arthritis who took one ounce of fresh ginger a day had significant relief of arthritis symptoms. One ounce equals 28 grams or 7 teaspoons of fresh grated ginger. In such cases, it is probably easier to take one 255mg capsule of concentrated ginger (a common sized capsule) three times a day.

Is ginger safe?

Research has shown that ginger is very safe. Animals that have been given daily amounts of ginger equivalent to a person's consumption of about 7.5 pounds have not suffered any noticeable ill effects. As a precaution, however, do not take ginger if you have a high fever or have symptoms that indicate a "hot" condition: dehydration, dryness with a rapid pulse, red skin, a bright red tongue, or blood in the stool. Taking ginger may exacerbate these symptoms.

How important is the extraction process in ensuring that I get the best ginger extract?

According to the manufacturers of various ginger extract products which are produced using a patented extraction method, the process is critical in ensuring you receive a high-quality, potent product. There are several manufacturers who use their own special extraction and processing methods to produce ginger extract products, which can include capsules, liquid extract, and syrup.

When I buy a ginger supplement, how can I be sure I'm getting a good quality product?

When you read the label on a ginger supplement, look for those that say the contents are "standardized." This means that it is guaranteed by analysis to contain the proper amount of gingerols and shogaol. It is preferable to find a brand that states the level of gingerols.

What other things should I consider when purchasing a ginger extract?

Also important to the quality of the end product are the conditions under which the ginger is grown and harvested. Climate (as with wine, some years are better than others for a ginger crop), organic versus conventional growing, and harvesting methods affect the product you pick up from the shelves. This is information you can obtain from the manufacturer or any literature written about the product, preferably by unbiased users or researchers.

Where can I get ginger extracts?

Ginger extracts are available through health food stores, pharmacies, natural food stores, mail order, and over the Internet. There are several high-quality products on the market. As with any supplement or remedy, learn as much about it before you take it. See appendix B for a list of sources of ginger extract products, including Zinaxin.

Can I get any benefit from adding ginger to my recipes?

The amount of ginger included in food recipes is usually not sufficient to cure any specific medical condition. But even a small amount of ginger in your diet can enhance any ginger supplements you are taking, plus have a preventive role in your health. If nothing else, cooking with ginger can improve absorption of nutrients, prevent food poisoning, and promote digestion.

❖
EIGHT
❖

The Controversy:
Does MSM Really Work?

Whenever a new supplement, drug, or other health-related product is introduced to the marketplace, especially one that has the potential to improve the lives of millions of people, there is a flood of information about the item from several sources. Those with many positive things to say include the developers and manufacturers of the product, as well as medical professionals and scientists who have observed its positive effects. Another group with good things to say are the patients themselves who have enjoyed the product's benefits.

Then there are the people who approach the idea with caution, wanting more studies and more evidence that the claims being made are valid. Far from being "doomsdayers," these people offer a different perspective and a "braking" system to the sometimes runaway enthusiasm projected by the first group.

Finally, there are those individuals who have little or nothing good to say about the product. This group may include anyone whose business may be hurt by the success (real or not) of the new product, as well as researchers who truly believe the agent does not live up to the claims and patients who have experienced either no benefit or have been harmed by the product.

MSM draws commentary from all categories. In this chapter, you will learn the pros and cons of what the research shows, what physicians report about their clinical experiences, and what patients say about their personal experiences with MSM. Also discussed are ways MSM may work toward the relief of arthritis symptoms with other natural remedies, such as chondroitin, glucosamine, various vitamins and minerals, and other nutrients.

EARLY CLINICAL FINDINGS ABOUT MSM

The pioneers of MSM research, Stanley Jacob, M.D., and Robert Herschler, M.D., began their work with the organic sulfur as an outgrowth of their research of DMSO, a chemical similar to

MSM. In 1963, Drs. Jacob and Herschler reported that DMSO was effective in the treatment of joint and muscle pain, rheumatoid arthritis, skin ulcers, psoriasis, bursitis, emphysema, and interstitial cystitis (a painful chronic bladder infection). In 1983, when both doctors were working at the Department of Surgery, Oregon Health Sciences University, in Portland, they reported on the state of research of DMSO and made some prophetic comments about MSM.

What did Drs. Jacob and Herschler say?

Based on the research and clinical studies they had conducted thus far, the doctors said there was one by-product of DMSO that appeared to have potential commercial value. That by-product was a stable metabolite of DMSO referred to as methylsulfonylmethane, or MSM. They predicted that MSM would gain significant worldwide attention as a dietary supplement, because their work indicated that most people are deficient in this necessary mineral.

What kind of research did Drs. Jacob and Herschler do on MSM?

Yes. From that point, the doctors conducted years of laboratory research and clinical trials using MSM in both animals and humans for a wide variety of medical conditions. Dr. Jacob treated more than 15,000 patients for a wide variety of medical conditions. He gave them doses of 250 to 750 mg per day, and occasionally doses as high as 5,000 mg per day, and reported excellent therapeutic results without side effects.

Dr. Herschler documented study after study as he prepared the way for what eventually resulted in eleven patents for various applications for MSM. Like the work conducted by Dr. Jacob and his research team, the results obtained by Dr. Herschler were impressive. Overall, both investigators found that MSM was effective in the treatment of many disorders and symptoms, including the pain and inflammation associated with arthritis and rheumatoid disorders; skin disorders such as acne, wrinkles, and dryness; gastrointestinal disorders, especially those associated with allergies and ingesting aspirin and other NSAIDs; chronic constipation; snoring; allergic reactions to environmental, food, and drug allergens, as well as allergy-induced asthma; muscle cramps, including nocturnal leg cramps and muscle spasms; and a wide range of parasite-related illnesses.

What are doctors today saying about MSM?

Physicians around the country have been trying MSM, prescribing it for their patients as well as using it for their own symptoms. One common thread among doctors who use MSM in their practices is that it is one of several supplements or remedies in their arsenals. Arnold Fox, M.D., president of the American Association of Pain Management and author of numerous books, including *Immune for Life* and *The Healthy Prostate*, recommends MSM for his patients who have arthritis. While he has found MSM to be helpful for this condition, he notes that he and physicians like him "use so many different things that it's hard to attribute success to any one particular substance." In the case of arthritis, these other substances can include glucosamine sulfate, chondroitin sulfate, ginger, antioxidants, essential fatty acids, and other nutrients.

Other physicians echo his sentiments. Steven J. Bock, M.D., co-director of Rhinebeck Health Center for Progressive Medicine in New York, as well as clinical instructor at Albany Medical College, often prescribes MSM for his patients with arthritis, as well as ginger extracts, glucosamine sulfate, and chondroitin sulfate. He believes that finding the right combination of natural remedies for each patient is key to successful therapy, and that MSM plays an important part in treatment for arthritis sufferers.

Hunter Yost, M.D., a orthomolecular physician in Tucson, Arizona, treats many patients who come to him with various allergies, autoimmune disorders, chronic fatigue, and arthritis. If, after testing a patient for levels of various nutrients, he detects a need for sulfur, MSM is included as part of a therapeutic program that consists of several other elements.

Marcellus Walker, M.D., who practices in Honesdale, Pennsylvania, notes that most people "really do need sulfur," and also believes "that it would work better in conjunction with other minerals. Most people are mineral deficient, too." Indeed, the very nature of the human body and the fact that so many elements must work together to accomplish specific tasks indicates that if you are deficient in one element you are likely deficient in others. Taking MSM to provide the sulfur that is so lacking in nearly everyone's diet appears to be a safe, natural, and healthy thing to do.

As one researcher put it, for some people taking MSM may be like putting high-octane gas into a car that is low on brake fluid, has an oil leak, and has one flat tire: they've paid good attention to one area but the car still won't run well until they remedy the other problems. Because of the synergistic nature of the human body, achieving and maintaining a balance of its essential nutrients is a key to good health, and, say physicians, should be considered anytime individual supplements are added to your diet.

What are doctors saying about MSM and arthritis in particular?

Many doctors, including Dr. Marcellus Walker, believe that people with arthritis have an accumulation of toxins in their joints, which is one cause of their pain and inflammation. MSM can provide relief to these patients because it helps eliminate the toxins from the body. To stimulate the detoxification process, high levels of MSM are needed. Dr. Jacob found that high doses of MSM—2,000 to 5,000 mg per day for 2 to 4 weeks, along with comparable amounts of vitamin C—were very effective in reducing the pain, inflammation, and swelling experienced by people with arthritis. These dosages are typical of those used for detoxification. A physician in New Jersey uses up to 10,000 mg per day for 7 to 10 days for people with severe crippling arthritis and notes "dramatic realignment and good health." Dr. Bock notes similar results using 8,000 to 10,000 mg per day in his patients with severe arthritis.

What are some reasons why MSM may not help?

Not every person who has tried MSM has experienced the results he or she wanted. This is to be expected, especially since it appears that many of the people who are using MSM are doing so on their own, with little or no advice or guidance from a health-care practitioner. The following reasons why MSM may not have helped some individuals are based on comments from people who tried MSM and were disappointed: (1) they weren't patient and quit using it too soon; (2) they took too high a dose and had a negative reaction (see the question in chapter 9 about ill effects and detoxification); (3) they didn't take enough and didn't bother to increase the dose to see if that made a difference. There are probably other reasons, including the fact that some people may not need supplemental sulfur, but these three appear to be the primary ones.

WHAT DO MSM USERS HAVE TO SAY?

The real test of the culmination of research and endless studies is whether a product delivers what it claims and that it does so with utmost safety—and, preferably, convenience and affordability as well. Based on anecdotal reports from people across the country, many men, women, and children are experiencing good to excellent results while they use MSM.

• A twenty-three-year-old man in Connecticut had suffered with acne for more than seven years. To control it, he had taken tetracycline every day for nearly five years. In desperation, he decided to try MSM. After going off the tetracycline for one week, he took 2,000 mg MSM, divided into two doses, for three days. The acne disappeared, and he continues to take a maintenance dose of 1,000 mg a day.

• A chronic case of athlete's foot is under control thanks to several applications of MSM lotion every week. The patient, a forty-four-year-old construction worker, had chronic athlete's foot because he needed to wear heavy socks and work boots every day on the job. He tried several over-the-counter powders and sprays and finally resorted to going to a dermatologist, who prescribed terbinafine. The fungus finally cleared up, only to return when he stopped using the medication. Tired of the expense and of having to apply the medication every day, he decided to try MSM lotion. After only one week of applying MSM every day, he stopped the terbinafine and is now able to keep the problem away by applying MSM lotion between his toes only twice a week.

• Three women coworkers, all of whom experienced cramps, headache, and occasional hot flashes premenstrually, decided to try MSM. One of the three women often had at least one day per month when she felt too ill to work. All three women reported a significant reduction in PMS symptoms, and the one woman who had often missed work hasn't missed a day since starting MSM.

• A thirty-year-old woman who had had bleeding gums for more than six months decided to try brushing her gums with MSM powder after reading how sulfur is effective in removing plaque, which contributes to tooth decay and gum disease. After one week of brushing twice a day with MSM powder, her gums stopped bleeding, and they have remained healthy ever since.

• About 4 million people suffer with tendinitis, a type of arthritis that is caused by repetitive motion, usually related to sports or work. One example is tennis elbow, a condition that afflicted a forty-year-old tennis instructor in Arizona. To cope with the pain from the tendinitis, he took ibuprofen several times a day, but after about three months the medication wasn't working and he was experiencing a lot of pain during his tennis classes. When a friend told him about MSM, he was skeptical but knew he needed to try something. He started at 1,000 mg a day for three days, then increased to 2,000 mg and increased a little every few days until he reached 6,000 mg a day after three weeks. At week two he felt about 50 percent better, and by week six, he was experiencing no pain. He still takes MSM at a maintenance dose of 750 mg per day and increases it to 2,000 or 3,000 whenever he overworks the arm or feels pain.

• Many people with adult onset diabetes are prescribed insulin or oral drugs by their doctors and are still unable to regulate their sugar levels. Such was the case with a fifty-two-year-old woman in Washington who was taking oral hypoglycemic drugs. Although she was careful with her food and exercise program, she had trouble controlling her sugar levels. She often felt fatigued, and her concern over her inability to control her sugar only made her feel worse. After reading about MSM, she asked her doctor if she could take it while still taking her medications. After one week she noticed her sugar levels were evening out, even though she had not changed anything else in her life. By three months, she had weaned herself off her oral hypoglycemia drugs and was taking 1,500 mg MSM per day. She has stayed at that level, feels energetic, and plans to take MSM indefinitely.

• A long-distance runner living in Colorado was

experiencing muscle soreness while training for a marathon. This twenty-nine-year-old woman was careful about stretching both before and after her training sessions, but the soreness persisted, and it was affecting her ability to recover after a workout. She was not in pain and did not want to use an analgesic or anti-inflammatory because of the potential side effects. A fellow runner told her about MSM, and she began to take 2,000 mg before her daily runs. She noticed some improvement, but when she increased the dosage to 3,000 she felt 100 percent better. She has maintained the 3,000mg daily dose and reports that she doesn't experience the cramped muscles she occasionally had before using MSM.

• Recurring constipation was the problem for a forty-one-year-old woman in New Jersey. She did experience some improvement after adding more fiber to her diet and drinking more water, yet she could expect at least one day of constipation per week, and several days of it when her period started. She began taking 1,000 mg MSM daily and after only two weeks noticed the constipation had not returned. The real test came when it was time for her period, but again the constipation did not occur.

• A thirty-year-old woman who works as a word processor for a large marketing firm had developed carpal tunnel syndrome. Despite wearing a wrist brace, redesigning her workstation, and taking ibuprofen daily, the pain was not well controlled. When her doctor suggested surgery, she knew she needed another option. A co-worker told her about MSM, and she began both taking an oral dose, 3,000 mg per day, and applying an MSM cream to her wrists. The improvement was gradual, and after four weeks she had reduced her twice daily intake of ibuprofen down to once every other day.

• Heartburn plagued a forty-seven-year-old Florida man who popped antacids like they were candy. His doctor convinced him to stop eating acidic foods, such as citrus and tomatoes, and to eliminate alcohol almost completely, yet the pain and reflux continued. For more than six months he switched back and forth between taking Zantac and Pepcid, which was harming his stomach and causing him to suffer with headaches. Then his wife read about MSM and bought it for him. After three weeks of taking both MSM and Zantac, he noticed a significant reduction in the incidence of heartburn. He stopped taking the Zantac and continued with 2,000 mg MSM a day—1,000 in the morning and 1,000 at night. As long as he continues with the MSM, he is both heartburn- and headache-free.

• A sixteen-year-old girl in Virginia had been tested for allergens at the age of six and was found to be allergic to a laundry list of items, including dust, animal hair, various pollens, grasses, and mold. After undergoing a series of shots over a two-year period beginning at age seven, she improved slightly for several years, but as she entered puberty the allergies seemed to come back stronger. She and her mother did not want to depend on antihistamines, so they turned to herbal remedies, including echinacea and goldenseal. She had moderate improvement: her sneezing spells decreased and her runny nose and itchy eyes improved, yet she still suffered enough so that she was often uncomfortable and had to stay indoors much of the time. When a friend suggested MSM, she started taking 1,000 mg in the morning and again in the evening, along with the herbs. After only three days of taking MSM, her symptoms had nearly vanished. As long as she continues to take MSM, she is symptom-free. If she forgets to take it for a few days, she is reminded by the return of itchy eyes and sneezing to take the MSM.

• A seventy-four-year-old grandmother in California who was once very active in her community was now limited because of arthritis. She had given up her folk dance classes because of the pain in her legs and hip and struggled with her gardening on her "good days." Her doctor had prescribed diclofenac, which was not very effective, and which left her constipated, often with stomach distress. Her neighbor was taking MSM for arthritis and recommended it to her. She started with 1,000 mg twice a day and gradually increased it to 3,000 mg twice a day. After one month she was able to garden again with very little discomfort. At two months, she rejoined her dance class. She has continued with the MSM, has stopped the diclofenac, and supplements with ibuprofen as needed. An additional benefit is that she no longer suffers with chronic constipation or stomach discomfort.

❧

NINE

❧

MSM and Other Medical Conditions

The healing qualities of MSM do not begin and end with arthritis and rheumatic disorders. Dr. Jacob and his research team have administered MSM to more than 15,000 patients over the years and documented how it has worked for a wide variety of medical conditions. Similarly, Dr. Herschler conducted endless clinical studies for his work on the patents for MSM, studies that covered a range of medical problems. Overall, both researchers report excellent results of their investigations.

Based largely on the work of these two investigators, other doctors across the United States and around the world have incorporated MSM into their practices. This chapter reports on the different diseases and medical conditions for which MSM has been used and the results of those treatments.

ALLERGIES

Dr. Herschler has had personal experience with the anti-allergy properties of MSM. After he found that taking MSM allowed him to forgo the antihistamines he had previously needed to control three different allergies he experienced every year, he conducted animal trials to confirm his own observations. He found that MSM provides relief from the allergic reactions to specific foods, drugs, and environmental substances.

What is an allergic reaction?

An allergic reaction is the immune system's combat response to substances known as allergens. To fight off these unwanted elements, the body produces antibodies, which cling to cells in the gastrointestinal and respiratory tracts. There the antibodies release various chemicals, including histamine, which is the culprit that causes allergic reactions. Allergic reactions, which can include sneezing, watery eyes, sore throat, ear infection, rash or hives, stuffy nose and head, stomach cramps, headache, urinary frequency, fatigue, diarrhea, and sometimes even asthma, are the body's way of trying to get rid of something it perceives as foreign and invasive.

What are the different types of allergies?

People can have allergic reactions to three general types of allergens: environmental, food, and medical (drugs). Environmental allergens include pollen, dust, mold, wool, mildew, dander, smoke, exhaust, perfume, pesticides, cosmetics, cleaning products, paints, glues, dyes, carpeting, and many other common items. Common food allergies include wheat, eggs, citrus, yeast, peanuts, dairy products, and seafood. Allergic reactions to drugs are commonly seen with oral antibiotics, aspirin, and NSAIDs.

How does MSM prevent allergic reactions?

In essence, MSM prohibits allergens from bonding to the gastrointestinal tract, which in turn prevents them from causing allergic reactions. MSM is also useful in relieving any inflammation caused by allergic reactions.

More specifically, the presence of enough sulfur in the body enables the cell walls to pass foreign substances and toxins out of the body. When sulfur levels are low, cell walls become stiff and unyielding, and the allergens cannot escape.

How can I use MSM to prevent allergic reactions?

Dr. Jacob reports that people with food allergies had significantly less reaction after taking daily dosages of 100 to 1,000 mg MSM. Similar dosages were effective in eliminating or dramatically reducing allergic response to drugs.

To help eliminate allergens from your body, Earl Mindell, R. Ph., Ph.D., author of *Earl Mindell's Vitamin Bible*, among other works, recommends beginning the process by taking at least 6,000 mg of MSM per day for three weeks and then reducing the dosage to 3,000 mg. Along with the MSM he suggests taking 2,000 mg or more of vitamin C, increasing water intake, and including 250 mg pantothenic acid (vitamin B_5) and 250 to 500 mg quercetin to your daily supplement program until your symptoms are eliminated. Quercetin is a bioflavonoid that can decrease allergic reactions and inhibit inflammation.

Can I stop taking other allergy medications if I take MSM?

The answer to this question depends on the severity of your allergy or allergies. Most people can at least significantly reduce the amount of any antiallergy medication they are taking, while some can eliminate it completely. Reports from people who have hay fever or allergic asthma show that they achieve good control of their symptoms with only 25 percent of their previous medication.

My son is nine years old and has allergies. Is he too young to take MSM?

MSM is safe for adults and children, and is especially helpful for people with allergies, asthma, and hay fever. One mother reports that her young son (who weighs 55 pounds) had serious allergies and was very miserable, even with the medication prescribed by the doctor. Once he started to take MSM, he was able to stop the medication and has not had allergy symptoms as long as he takes MSM.

Dr. Herschler himself can vouch for the effectiveness of MSM in the treatment of allergies. Having suffered with respiratory allergies for year, he took MSM and got relief. When he stopped taking MSM, his symptoms returned.

DIABETES

Diabetes is characterized by faulty metabolism that results in excess blood glucose (sugar) and either no or poor production of insulin, or cell resistance to insulin. Approximately 16 million people in the United States have diabetes; half are undiagnosed. Of the two main types of diabetes, non-insulin dependent diabetes (NIIDD) is the more common. It usually first appears in people 40 years and older and makes up about 90 percent of all cases of diabetes. The other type, insulin-dependent diabetes, typically first appears in childhood and comprises about 5 to 10 percent of all diabetes cases.

What role does sulfur play in diabetes?

Sulfur is an especially important mineral for people with diabetes because it aids in carbohydrate metabolism and the utilization of glucose. A deficiency of dietary sulfur in people with diabetes can lead to reduced production of insulin and an increase in blood sugar levels, resulting in potentially dangerous medical conditions for these patients. Some diabetics are able to decrease their need for insulin injections when they increase their intake of sulfur.

Some experts believe that diabetes causes the cell walls to become impermeable, which means insulin and blood sugar cannot enter the cells. When sugar cannot be absorbed by the cells, it floods the bloodstream and raises the blood sugar level. In an attempt to compensate for what the body senses as a lack of insulin, the pancreas works overtime to produce more insulin and eventually malfunctions.

How does MSM help people with diabetes?

Supplementation with MSM may increase the permeability of cells, thus allowing insulin and sugar to pass through the cell walls. This results in a balance of blood sugar levels, and the pancreas may return to normal functioning.

What is the recommended dosage of MSM for people with type II diabetes?

Dr. Mindell recommends a minimum of 2,000 mg per day. Patients are urged to work with their physicians to determine the optimal dosage for their needs.

GASTROINTESTINAL COMPLAINTS

Problems with the gastrointestinal tract—which includes the esophagus, stomach, and large and small intestines—are common among people of all ages. Diarrhea and constipation are two of the most common health complaints; nausea, heartburn, and hyperacidity (excess acid in the stomach) are also high on the list. Oral doses of MSM have been successful in relieving these and other gastrointestinal problems.

arrhea?

haracterized by frequent bowel
d is usually caused by bacteria in
food, water. Most cases of diarrhea can be
cured in two to three days, although sometimes
diarrhea is an indication of an underlying condition, such as gastroenteritis. Gastroenteritis,
which is an infection and inflammation of the
gastrointestinal tract, affects more than 25 million people a year. Diarrhea may also indicate
irritable bowel syndrome, Crohn's disease, coli-
tis, lactose intolerance, or a reaction to a magnesium supplement. Chronic or long-term (more
than three days) diarrhea can cause dehydration
and should be treated professionally, especially
when it occurs in infants and the elderly.

Why is chronic constipation so common?

A poor diet—one that is low in fiber, high in
fat and/or sugar, and supported with insufficient water intake—is a major cause of constipation. Inadequate nutrition is then too-often
combined with other factors, such as high stress,
lack of physical exercise, the presence of other
medical conditions, and the use of medications
and even nutritional supplements may all contribute to chronic constipation. Many diuretics
and decongestants, for example, cause constipation, as do many iron supplements.

How can MSM help cure diarrhea and constipation?

Dr. Jacob has had success treating chronic constipation at a dose of 100 to 500 mg MSM a day. One study involved patients with chronic constipation taking 500 mg MSM along with 1,000 mg vitamin C per day. All patients were cured and remained constipation-free while they included MSM as part of their supplement program. To maintain good elimination habits and avoid constipation, include more fiber in your diet (fruits, vegetables, whole-grain products, beans) and drink at least eight glasses of water a day. If you are taking medications, check with your doctor to see if any of them may be causing constipation.

According to Dr. Jacob, most people who get diarrhea respond to 100 to 500 mg MSM daily. Dr. Mindell suggests starting with 3,000 mg.

What is heartburn?

The commercials about stomach acid make you think that the natural juices your stomach produces are a bad thing. Without stomach acid, however, and certain enzymes, you would not be able to break down your food properly and digest it. The stomach makes hydrochloric acid, which breaks down food, kills bad bacteria and parasites, and helps the body absorb nutrients.

The enzyme pepsin, which breaks down proteins, is also produced in the stomach. If the stomach doesn't make enough hydrochloric acid, food will remain in the stomach for hours. The result is heartburn—stomach pain and the sensation that food is coming back up into your throat, which is called acid reflux or gastroesophageal reflux.

Why do so many people have heartburn?

According to the National Institute of Diabetes and Digestive and Kidney Diseases, about 61 million American men and women experience heartburn at least once a month, and approximately 25 million have heartburn every day. Given the high stress levels and poor diet of many Americans, these high numbers are not unexpected. Unfortunately, most people quickly reach for one or more of the antacids or acid blockers on the market, either as a preventive measure or after the irritation has begun. Chronic use of these drugs can cause a long list of problems, including permanent damage of the natural acid/alkaline balance (pH) of the body.

Are antacids and acid blockers the same? What are they designed to do?

Antacids are over-the-counter medications designed to treat excess acid in the upper gastrointestinal tract, which includes the stomach and esophagus. Specifically, they neutralize some of the hydrochloric acid in the stomach and reduce the activity of a digestive enzyme called pepsin. There are dozens of antacids on the market with about two dozen different formulations. Some common antacids include Di-Gel, Gaviscon, Gelusil, Maalox, Mylanta, Riopan, and Tums.

Acid blockers, also known as histamine-H2 receptor antagonists, include both over-the-counter and prescription medications designed to treat duodenal and gastric ulcers and other conditions in which excess hydrochloric acid is a problem, and to treat and prevent heartburn. Rather than neutralize acid, acid blockers prohibit the release of a substance called histamine, and the result is less acid secreted by the stomach. Common generic and trade name acid blockers include cimetidine (Peptol, Tagamet), famotidine (Pepcid), and ranitidine (Zantac).

Both antacids and acid blockers provide only temporary relief of heartburn and excess acidity. Over time, these drugs can make these symptoms worse rather than better.

What kinds of side effects can antacids and acid blockers cause?

Occasional use of antacids usually does not cause problems. A few people experience mild constipation or a mild laxative effect, increased thirst, or stomach cramps. Similar use of acid blockers cause dizziness, headache, diarrhea, or diminished sex drive.

Unfortunately, many people use antacids and acid blockers every day or nearly every day. Chronic use of antacids can cause liver and kidney damage, malabsorption of B vitamins and minerals, and indigestion. Antacids that contain calcium carbonate can actually cause the stomach to produce more acid after you get some initial relief, and antacids that contain aluminum can cause constipation. Long-term use of acid blockers may damage the liver and cause severe headache, mental confusion, an inflamed pancreas, vomiting, and diarrhea.

How can MSM help heartburn and acidity?

Studies by Dr. Jacob show that MSM can provide fast, effective relief from heartburn and excess acidity without causing side effects. MSM appears to be safe enough to take every day, as it does not upset the pH balance or any other body functions. The average dose for heartburn is up to 750 mg per day, but Dr. Jacob has used up to 2,000 mg daily for 6 months in some patients without ill effects. Dr. Mindell suggests starting with a dosage of 3,000 mg.

Along with taking MSM for heartburn, consider the following lifestyle changes:

1. Avoid eating close to bedtime or lying down after you eat. Gravity causes acid to enter the esophagus.

2. Avoid fatty or fried foods, alcohol, chocolate, tomatoes and tomato products, spicy foods, citrus fruits and juices, and coffee.

3. Do not smoke.

4. Eat smaller meals more frequently and/or reduce the size of your meals. You are more likely to get heartburn when your stomach is full.

LUPUS

Systemic lupus erythematosus (SLE) is a form of arthritis in which the inflammation often affects the internal organs. It can be especially dangerous if it affects the heart, lungs, kidneys, and gastrointestinal tract.

What causes lupus?

Researchers know that lupus is an autoimmune disease, but they do not know what causes it. Several observations about who gets lupus may help investigators discover the cause. It is believed hormones play a part in development of the disease, as do age, sex, and genetics. Lupus is more prevalent among women of child-bearing age and among blacks. About 10 percent of first-degree relatives of people with lupus develop the disease, and there is a high prevalence among identical twins.

What are the symptoms of lupus?

Symptoms vary widely among patients with lupus, but the three most common ones are fever, arthritis, and rash. Exposure to the sun frequently triggers the rash, which may appear on the face across the nose and cheeks. General fatigue and weight loss are other common symptoms. In addition to joint pain and stiffness, some lupus patients develop inflammation of the lining that surrounds the lungs, heart, and abdomen, which can cause breathing difficulties. Some patients develop inflammation of the kidneys, bone marrow, or brain, all of which are potentially life-threatening conditions.

Can MSM be beneficial for people with lupus?

MSM can relieve the symptoms of joint pain, inflammation, and stiffness as it does for other forms of arthritis. So far, no specific investigations of its use in people with lupus have been conducted, although several studies have been done in animals with promising results.

MUSCLE SPASMS AND CRAMPS

Individuals who are susceptible to muscle spasms and cramps include the elderly, athletes, and anyone who experiences long sessions of standing or inactivity. MSM has proved useful in relieving the pain and discomfort associated with these symptoms.

How does MSM work to relieve muscle soreness, spasms, and cramps?

The muscles are rich with pain-sensitive nerves. When muscles become fatigued, stressed, or overworked, the pressure outside the cells falls. If your body does not have a sufficient supply of sulfur, the cells walls will be unable to allow fluids to pass freely through them to balance the uneven pressure between the outside of the cells and the inside. The result: the cells swell, causing the nerve cells to send message of pain to your brain. MSM restores flexibility to the cells by opening up the passage of fluids through their walls.

My husband has been experiencing leg cramps at night. Can MSM relieve them?

Dr. Herschler reported that "methylsulfonyl-methane has the surprising ability to reduce the incidence of or eliminate entirely muscle cramps ... particularly in geriatric patients who experience such cramps at night." Results are especially good when MSM is combined with equal amounts of vitamin C. This combination is also very effective in eradicating muscle spasms and back cramps. You can begin with a standard dosage of 250 to 750 mg and adjust as needed.

I take aerobics classes and work out with free weights at the gym. Can MSM help relieve my sore muscles or prevent them from getting fatigued?

When you work your muscles hard, the body builds up a supply of lactic acid in your cells. If your sulfur supply is low, the lactic acid and other toxins cannot leave your cells, and your muscles become sore. MSM inhibits lactic acid from accumulating and crystallizing and then flushes it out of the body. You can take MSM before your workouts to prevent soreness and immediately after to reduce the risk of cramping. Athletes report getting excellent results when taking 1,000 to 2,000 mg of MSM in 2 doses per day for 6 months.

PARASITE INFECTIONS

It is a common misconception that parasites exist only in poor, undeveloped countries that have sanitation problems, or that only barefoot farmers can contract these infections. Parasites may be a bigger problem than you think.

How common are parasite infections in the United States?

Experts estimate that 85 percent of Americans have at least one parasite in their body. These worms, which can range from microscopic amoeba to tapeworms measuring 30 feet or more, are the cause of many diseases and medical conditions in the United States. The American gastrointestinal tract harbors more than 130 different kinds of parasites, any one or more of which could travel through your bloodstream and attack your joints, organs, and muscles.

What kinds of illnesses and symptoms can be caused by internal parasites?

Parasites can cause a variety of conditions that are often misdiagnosed simply because many doctors are unfamiliar or untrained in parasitology. Common symptoms that can be attributed to parasites include unexplained gas or bloating, heart pain, blurred vision, unexplained muscular pain, cold or numb hands, chronic fatigue, loss of sex drive, depression, loss of appetite, overeating, unexplained menstrual problems, itching, and burning sensation in the stomach.

Why have parasites becomes so prevalent in the United States?

Parasites have become a problem for several reasons. One is that Americans are traveling abroad much more often and frequently. Along with vacation and business travelers, this includes our armed services personnel, missionaries, and relief volunteers. Other sources of parasites are the importation of exotic foods, especially fresh fruits and vegetables; contamination of the water supply; increased sexual contact; the increasing pet population; the large number of immigrants that arrive from parasite-infested regions of the world; rising use of day care facilities; and the use of immunosuppressive drugs.

Parasites remain prevalent once they make themselves at home in their victims because few people realize they are infected. Until they are diagnosed and eradicated, they will remain in the body, reproducing and causing health problems that affected individuals cannot explain.

What kinds of parasites can MSM eliminate from the body?

In Dr. Herschler's studies, he has shown that MSM has antiparasitic effects against various organisms, including nematodes, *Trichomonas*, *Giardia lamblia* (causes giardiasis), *Enterobius*, and other intestinal worms. MSM has the ability to allow the tissues affected by the parasites to heal without causing any harmful effects to the body.

How does MSM help rid the body of parasites?

Researchers believe MSM blocks any interaction between the parasites and the receptor sites on the mucous membranes to which parasites normally attach. When parasites cannot find a place to settle, they are eliminated through the intestinal tract.

How can I be tested for a parasitic infection?

Your doctor can administer several different stool, saliva, and blood tests, although you should know that some parasites are difficult to detect. Varying reproductive cycles and the tendency for some parasites to cling to the intestinal walls rather than show up in stool samples may mean you get a negative test result but may still have parasites in your system. Eosinophilia can usually be detected using a blood test.

How much MSM do I need to eliminate parasites from my body?

To start the cleansing process, Dr. Mindell recommends taking 10,000 mg of MSM every day for three to four weeks, then reducing the dosage to 3,000 mg. Lower doses have been shown to be effective as well: 750 to 1,500 mg per day, taken for 90 to 120 days, is often recommended. The dosage you need will depend on the extent of your infection.

What causes the symptoms associated with detoxification?

MSM is a negatively charged molecule, so it attracts positive molecules. Some of those molecules come from toxins that lurk in the body, such as mercury, lead, allergens, or other poisons from your food, water, or environment. These toxic substances can be eliminated from the body when you take MSM. This process of detoxification can cause some temporary problems, such as diarrhea, headache, fatigue, and rash. These are expected consequences of detoxification and typically last one to 10 days. If you have arthritis, as these toxins leave the body, so does arthritis pain, because these poisons accumulate in the joints and contribute to arthritis pain and inflammation. The same type of detoxification reaction can occur if you are trying to eliminate parasites, heavy metals, or other toxins from your body.

How much MSM do I need to take for the detoxification process?

Dr. Jacob and others generally prescribe 2,000 to 5,000 mg per day for several weeks and then reduce the dosage as the poisons leave the body. Some doctors use even higher dosages, up to 20,000 mg, for a short period of time, depending on the patient's needs.

The detoxification process that MSM causes sounds very beneficial, but how can I avoid the symptoms?

If you suspect you have heavy metal toxins or parasites in your system and want to avoid the toxic symptoms, begin with a lower dose of MSM; say, 750 mg twice a day. Gradually increase the dosage to 3,000 mg twice a day as tolerated. You may also want to consult with a health-care professional who is knowledgeable about MSM to determine your sulfur needs.

Are there any natural remedies I can take along with MSM to deal with parasite infections?

Several simple and safe remedies can be taken along with MSM. The herb goldenseal is a potent parasite killer, as is garlic, which you can either include in your diet or take as a supplement. Other herbs known for their antiparasitic ability are black walnut, mugwort, thyme, wormwood, and grapefruit seed extract. Follow the dosing directions on the package for these remedies.

SKIN AND NAIL CONDITIONS

Reports of the benefits MSM has on various skin problems have been very promising. Use of MSM in these areas has been well studied by both Drs. Jacob and Herschler.

How can MSM help erase wrinkles?

The body is constantly shedding old skin cells and replacing them with new ones. If you have a sulfur deficiency, the new cells will have cell walls that are impermeable and unyielding, which contributes to wrinkling. Supplementation with MSM can eventually provide your body with healthy new cells, and wrinkles will fade away.

I have scar tissue from surgery and stretch marks from childbirth. What can MSM do for me?

According to Dr. Herschler's patent information, MSM is effective in eliminating stretch marks, burns, surgical incisions, and other external marks and scar tissue. To treat these conditions, MSM is applied as a lotion, gel, or spray mist to the affected areas. When choosing a topical MSM product, select one that has as few artificial additives as possible, as these may cause adverse effects.

MSM also heals internal scars, which respond well to oral treatment, and accelerates wound healing.

Help! I have chronic athlete's foot. Can MSM help me?

An MSM lotion or gel can be used on the affected areas several times a week to stop the burning and itching and to eliminate the cracked skin between the toes. As a maintenance remedy, you may want to apply some lotion once a week. In chronic cases of athletes foot, taking 250 to 750 mg of MSM orally while also using topical MSM is beneficial.

My skin has always been very dry, and it's making me look older than I am. I've been using a lotion that contains collagen, but it doesn't seem to help. Can MSM help me?

MSM's role in keeping skin healthy is to keep the bonds between the skin cells flexible. It does this by preventing a process called cross-linking of collagen, which is associated with dry, tough, aging skin. If you have a deficiency of sulfur, the cells become rigid and the skin becomes dry, cracked, and wrinkled.

To help revitalize your skin and keep it supple and smooth, apply an MSM lotion daily to the skin and rub it in thoroughly. To feed your skin from the inside out, daily supplementation with MSM is recommended. Dr. Mindell suggests 1,000 mg with each meal.

If you use a skin product that contains collagen, you are wasting your time and money because the skin cannot absorb collagen. MSM taken internally stimulates the production of your body's own natural collagen and revives it.

Are there other natural substances I can take along with MSM to improve my skin?

Good skin care should include adequate levels of vitamins A, C, and E (therapeutic dosages: A, as beta-carotene, 25,000 IU; C, 2,000 mg; E, 800 IU). In addition, there are skin care products on the market that contain MSM and other revitalizing nutrients, such as aloe vera and antioxidant vitamins such as A, C, and E. See appendix B for suppliers.

Can people with scleroderma benefit from MSM?

Scleroderma is a potentially fatal disease in which the connective tissue hardens, shrinks, and tightens. It can be localized or spread throughout the body and affect the skin or any of the organs, including the heart, lungs, liver, esophagus, and kidneys. Older people are the most likely victims.

Both Drs. Jacob and Herschler found that application of topical MSM can relieve the tightness characteristic of this disease. MSM lotions, which contain about 15 percent MSM, are safe to use several times a day without concern for adverse effects.

What other skin conditions are relieved with MSM?

Dr. Herschler found that pruritis and acne respond well to oral supplements of 100 to 1,000 mg per day. To treat acne in teenagers, MSM was added to cola drinks and was more readily accepted.

If you are bothered by poison ivy or poison oak, applying MSM lotion to the affected areas reportedly eliminates the itch. Oral supplements (500 to 2,000 mg) are also helpful in relieving sunburn and neutralizing the toxins from insect bites.

OTHER USES FOR MSM

During the course of their research, Drs. Jacob and Herschler uncovered several other medical conditions and symptoms that may be eliminated or significantly alleviated with MSM. And humans are not the only ones who benefit from supplementation with MSM. In fact, MSM has been used to treat both livestock and domestic animals longer than it has been administered to people.

My husband snores so loud it keeps me awake at night. Can MSM help me get some sleep?

According to a study conducted at Oregon Health Sciences University, 8 to 16 drops of MSM (in a 16 percent water solution) administered in each nostril 10 to 60 minutes before bedtime for 90 days significantly reduced snoring in 80 percent of those treated. Subsequent studies, which used higher concentrations of MSM, had even better results.

I've suffered with chronic headaches for years. Should I try MSM?

Many people who experience chronic headache get relief when they take MSM daily. MSM appears to work best for headache caused by muscle tension, because it has the ability to ease muscle spasm. MSM also makes the cell walls more permeable, which in turn increases circulation, results in a drop in pressure, and reduces inflammation. Routine supplementation of MSM is recommended as a preventive measure to help maintain good circulation.

It is also suggested that you identify the causes of your head pain. Chronic physical and/or emotional stress, food allergies, environmental toxins, and possible contributing medical problems should be considered when treating headache pain. In most cases, MSM can be a major factor in providing relief.

I've seen MSM eyedrops on the market. What eye problems can be helped with MSM?

When the tissues in the eye are healthy, they allow the free passage of fluids through the membrane wall of the eyeball. This membrane filters out damaging particles and allows nutrients to enter. If the membrane becomes rigid, the particles become trapped in the eyeball, and cataracts form.

Use of a 15 percent eyedrop solution of MSM can help return permeability to the membrane. Dr. Jacob reports that MSM is excellent for treatment of eye infections, conjunctivitis, and glaucoma. It is also important to note that healthy eyes require adequate levels of B vitamins, the sulfur amino acids, glucosamine, and glutathione (see chapter 6).

What benefits can I expect from using MSM toothpaste and mouthwash?

In a test that compared regular commercial toothpaste with a tooth powder mixed 50/50 with MSM, all signs of gum inflammation disappeared after one week in subjects who used the MSM powder. Researchers also noted the disappearance of canker sores in one subject and an improved sense of smell in two individuals who had previously had a limited sense of smell.

Can MSM improve my mental state or level of concentration?

It's been observed among people who have taken MSM that their level of awareness and alertness improves and their frequency of depression is low. Students who use MSM say their ability to concentrate is enhanced. Some depressed individuals who take MSM report that they get relief within hours instead of within days as they do when using antidepressants alone.

Has MSM shown any promise in treating people with Alzheimer's disease?

There are a few anecdotal reports that MSM has helped restore memory in people with Alzheimer's disease. The claims from family members are that MSM removed aluminum from the brain of patients. The cause of Alzheimer's disease is not known, and aluminum toxicity is a controversial area. Therefore use of MSM for this form of dementia remains highly speculative.

I've heard that MSM can help the terminally ill. How is it used for these individuals?

MSM is given to terminally ill patients to help establish what is known as mental normalcy, which is a state of alertness and inner calmness without a tendency to experience mood swings or marked depression. To ease anxiety and depression in dying patients, Dr. Mindell suggests administering up to 9,000 mg per day and then gradually reducing the dosage to 3,000 mg per day.

If MSM is so good for people, can my pets benefit, too?

Use of MSM by veterinarians has been well established for many years. Much of the pioneering work with DMSO and MSM was done in horses, and what was learned is very appropriate for smaller companion animals as well. If you want to promote general good health and shiny coats for your dogs, cats, and horses, you can give them an MSM supplement each day. Depending on the size of cat or dog, mix ⅛ to ¼ teaspoon MSM powder into their food daily. For horses, use 1 to 2 tablespoons daily.

MSM has many other uses for companion animals, horses, and livestock, especially in the treatment of arthritis, wounds, lung disorders, intestinal problems, and skin conditions. Talk with your veterinarian about these uses.

TEN

❦

Buying and Using MSM

You've read how MSM is a natural nutritional supplement that performs many essential functions in the body. You've learned how it can help improve many aspects of your health and well-being. Now all that's left is buying and using MSM. Before you start taking MSM, or any supplement, it is best to consult with your physician and let him or her know about any medications or other remedies you may be taking. Do not reduce the amount of any medication you are taking without first talking with your physician. These safety measures can prevent the occurrence of unforeseen side effects or adverse reactions.

Where can I buy MSM?

MSM is available in the supplement section of most pharmacies, drugstores, and natural food stores, and even some supermarkets. You can also get it from nutritionists, from naturopaths, and by mail order (see appendix A).

In what forms is MSM available?

You can purchase MSM in several forms to accommodate your preferences and the different conditions you may need to treat: capsules, each usually containing 100 to 500 mg MSM; powder, which can be dissolved in any nonalcoholic liquid or mixed with food; and as a lotion, gel, or spray mist for topical applications to treat pain and swelling. MSM is also available in eyedrops, for eye disease, infections, and inflammation; and as a toothpaste, for gum disease and general dental hygiene.

What are the advantages of using capsules over powder?

Capsules are convenient and easy to carry with you. People who are taking lower doses of MSM, usually defined as 3,000 mg or less, find that the 500mg capsules make dosing easy. For people who are taking higher doses, especially 8,000 mg or more, the idea of taking 16 or more capsules a day is unappealing, so the powder is more convenient.

What's the best way to use MSM powder?

The powder is slightly bitter, so you may want to dissolve it in juice, coffee, or tea. Water is the best choice, however, and soda is not recommended because of its unhealthy sugar content. The powder dissolves best in warm or hot liquids. For dosing, 1 teaspoon equals 4 grams (¼ teaspoon equals 1 gram).

Which MSM topical solution is the best?

Topical MSM is available in lotion, gel, and cream. Some products contain only MSM mixed into a standard gel or lotion; others consist of MSM plus other ingredients, such as vitamin E. Topicals that contain MSM alone may be the better choice, as there is no evidence that combination products are any more effective.

How much MSM supplement should I take?

According to Dr. Herschler, the fact "that nearly everyone is sulfur deficient during part of each day surprises many." To ensure that the body has an adequate level of MSM at all times, he recommends 2,000 to 5,000 mg taken either once or twice each day. Dr. Jacob recommends about 2,000 mg a day for general health and maintenance, and higher doses for therapeutic purposes.

Dr. Earl Mindell suggests a daily maintenance or therapeutic dose of 2,000 to 6,000 mg. The truth is, the most beneficial dosage depends on your age, body size, your MSM blood level before beginning supplementation, and the severity of the condition you are treating, if any. Dr. Jacob has seen excellent response to MSM in people who take 250 to 750 mg per day, although some of the more than 15,000 patients he has treated have suffered no ill effects when taking doses up to 5,000 mg per day. It is believed the systemic concentration of MSM declines with age; therefore older individuals should take a dose that is in the higher range.

The best advice is to start with a low dose and gradually increase it over two to three weeks. For therapeutic purposes, start with 2,000 mg per day and increase 1,000 mg after a few days. Gradually increase the dose until you get a response.

Should I take the entire daily dose at once, or divide it over the course of the day?

Most health professionals recommend you take MSM in divided doses; for example, if you are taking 2,000 mg per day, take 1,000 at breakfast and 1,000 at dinner. This approach allows your body to get used to the MSM more easily and reduces the possibility of gastrointestinal problems. Also, it is best to take MSM three to four hours before you retire, because some people report feeling very energetic after taking MSM, which can disrupt your sleep cycle.

Should I take MSM with food?

Although stomach problems are not a common occurrence among people who take MSM, it is best to take it during meals or after eating to minimize your chances of getting any type of gastrointestinal response. If you are using MSM powder, mixing it with your food makes dosing convenient.

Can I overdose on MSM?

There is some debate about whether taking "too much" MSM can cause ill effects or toxicity. Many researchers claim that MSM is no more toxic than ordinary water. Others, like George Bergstrom of Cardinal Associates Marketing, manufacturers of MSM, caution that temporary stomach upset may occur in people who take more than 5,000 mg per day, which is the maximum dosage recommended by Dr. Jacob. Earl Mindell, author of *Earl Mindell's Vitamin Bible* and other books on nutrition, believes that "within limits, you cannot overdose with MSM," because 12 hours after taking the supplement, the body eliminates any excess amounts.

The key words here may be "within limits." According to Dr. Marcellus Walker, problems with MSM toxicity may arise in people who literally cannot "stomach" supplemental sulfur. That's because one of sulfur's abilities is to eliminate poisons from the body. People who have high levels of toxins in their system may suffer some ill effects when they take MSM because the liver dumps toxic bile into the stomach. A dose of MSM that causes gastrointestinal problems in a person who has high toxic levels may not have a bad impact on a person with low toxic levels. (Additional discussion of MSM and its role in detoxification appears in chapter 9.)

If you experience gastrointestinal problems, frequent stools, and/or minor headache when taking MSM, reduce your dose until these symptoms disappear.

How safe is MSM?

Overall, indications from years of short- and long-term studies indicate that MSM is very safe when taken at suggested doses. Drs. Jacob and Herschler conducted toxicity studies in both humans and animals to see if MSM causes toxic effects. All their results showed that MSM has a toxicity level similar to that of water. Thus in order for a dose to be lethal, an individual would have to consume a tremendous amount of MSM: a 110-pound woman, for example, would have to take more than 1,000 grams per day—that's equal to two thousand 500-mg capsules!

Some people have taken more than 100 grams of MSM a day (under a doctor's supervision) without experiencing any side effects. Yet the average daily dose ranges from as little as 750 mg up to 6 grams (or 6,000 mg) or more.

Not everyone completely agrees, however, that MSM is safe. John Cardellina, director of botanical sciences and editorial affairs at the Council for Responsible Nutrition in Washington, DC, is apprehensive about MSM and urges caution. "I'm hard pressed to think of any nutritive value of this stuff whatsoever," he says. He questions the validity of the studies on MSM, saying "we have not found anything resembling a clinical trial or a serious biological study under rationally designed conditions." He noted that he and his colleagues would likely conduct investigations into MSM to determine its safety.

How do I know how much MSM I need to take?

Questions about dosage are probably among the most asked about MSM. Throughout this book there are suggested dosages for MSM for arthritis (see chapter 5) and many other individual medical conditions and symptoms (see chapter 9). Because many people who use MSM are doing so on their own without professional supervision, they are often experimenting with dosages. It is best to consult with a health-care professional who can help you determine if you need sulfur and how much to take.

How quickly should I expect to get relief from pain?

This is a difficult question to answer because there are so many kinds of pain. One point to remember is that MSM is a nutrient and not a prescribed pain medication that kills pain within minutes. Although MSM does provide quick pain relief for many people, it works best on chronic pain conditions, such as arthritis, recurring headache, and fibromyalgia, because you can take it indefinitely without worrying about side effects.

Is there any way to boost the pain-relieving power of MSM?

Many people find that applying MSM lotion, cream, or gel to areas that are painful and/or inflamed, in addition to taking an oral dose, improves the amount of pain relief.

Is it safe to take prescription medications while taking MSM?

Throughout the many years of research and use of MSM in tens of thousands of patients, MSM has not been shown to have any negative effect on most prescription drugs. In fact, you may notice that you can reduce or even stop prescribed drugs once you are taking MSM regularly. Do not, however, stop taking any prescribed medication without first talking with your physician.

One possible interaction may occur between MSM and blood-thinning drugs such as aspirin, heparin, or dicumarol. Researchers note that MSM appears to have some blood-thinning abilities; thus if you take MSM while you are on known blood-thinners, there is a remote possibility you may experience bruising. Consult with your doctor before starting MSM if you are taking a blood thinner.

❁

Afterword:
The Future of MSM

What does the future hold for MSM? If the past and present are any indication, it is promising indeed. For those people who have used MSM and experienced relief from the symptoms of arthritis, heartburn, leg cramps, allergies, diarrhea, constipation, headache, and other medical conditions, the future is brighter. For those who have not yet tried MSM, the promise of relief is there.

MSM is not a cure-all. It is not for every symptom, every disease, or every illness, and it will not help everyone who tries it. But when taken as directed, this natural, safe nutrient may provide you or a loved one with much needed and thus far elusive relief from pain and discomfort.

❦

Glossary

Amino acids—organic acids that are the building blocks of proteins.

Analgesic—a drug that is taken to relieve pain but is not effective for inflammation; acetaminophen is an example.

Antioxidant—a substance that stops oxidation by attacking free radicals and preventing them from damaging cells and tissues.

Arthritis—a general term for about 100 diseases and related disorders which share the common characteristics of pain, inflammation, and limited movement of the joints.

Bioflavonoids—substances found in most plant foods that are necessary for the metabolism of vitamin C and for healthy capillaries.

Cartilage—the rubbery tissue that acts as a shock

absorber where the ends of the bones meet in a joint. Collagen is one of its main components.

Chondroitin sulfates—naturally occurring substances that prohibit the enzymes that can damage cartilage.

Coenzyme—a substance, usually a vitamin, that activates an enzyme.

Collagen—a protein that makes up the main component of connective tissue and the matrix in teeth and bones.

Enzyme—a substance that acts as a catalyst to initiate and speed up chemical reactions.

Essential fatty acid—a fatty acid that cannot be manufactured by the body and so must be supplied by the diet.

Free radicals—unstable molecules that are necessary for life but which can also cause damage by attracting electrons from other molecules.

Gastrointestinal—referring to the organs that comprise the digestive tract, from the mouth to the anus.

Glucosamine—a substance found naturally in the body that determines how many water-holding molecules are made in cartilage.

Glucose—a sugar found in the blood that is used for energy; also, a substance found in sugars and fruits that forms starch.

Keratin—a sulfur-containing protein found in hair, skin, and nails.

Macronutrients—nutrients the body needs in large amounts—proteins, carbohydrates, fats, and water.

Micronutrients—nutrients the body needs in smaller amounts, such as vitamins and minerals.

Minerals—inorganic substances that the body needs in small amounts for proper functioning.

NSAIDs—nonsteroidal anti-inflammatory drugs, which are usually taken to relieve pain and inflammation.

Organelles—various organ-like structures within cells.

Placebo—an inactive or dummy substance often used as a control in clinical studies.

Prednisone—an artificial cortisone drug used to treat inflammation and usually prescribed for people with rheumatoid arthritis.

Prostaglandins—hormone-like substances that have several functions in the body, including dilation of blood vessels and contraction of smooth muscle; they are responsible for inflammation.

Synovial fluid—a lubricating fluid found in the joints.

Uric acid—the byproduct of the metabolism of

purines, which are nonprotein substances. Excess uric acid is a sign of gout.

Vitamins—organic compounds that the body needs to function properly.

❀

Appendix A:
Souces of Information

ARTHRITIS

American Chronic Pain Association
P.O. Box 850
Rocklin, CA 95677
1-916-632-0922
e-mail: ACPA@pacbell.net

American College of Rheumatology
http://www.rheumatology.org
1-404-633-3777

Ankylosing Spondylitis Association
P.O. Box 5872
Sherman Oaks, CA 91413

1-800-777-8189
http://www.spondyl.org

Arthritis Consulting Services
4620 N. State Road, Suite 206
Fort Lauderdale, FL 33319
1-800-327-3027

The Arthritis Foundation
1330 West Peachtree St.
Atlanta GA 30309
800-283-7800
Also call your local chapter in the telephone directory.
http://www.arthritis.org

National Institute of Arthritis and Musculoskeletal and Skin Diseases
NIH Information Clearinghouse
1 AMS Circle
Bethesda, MD 20892-3675
301-495-4484; fax 301-587-4352
Also an online brochure on arthritis and exercise at http://www.nih.gov/niams/healthinfo/arthexfs.htm

National Institute on Aging
NIA Information Center
P.O. Box 8057

Gaithersburg, MD 20898-8057
1-800-222-2225; or e-mail
   niainfo@access.digex.net
for free publications

STRESS MANAGEMENT

The Academy for Guided Imagery
P.O. Box 2070
Mill Valley, CA 94942
1-800-726-2070

American Board of Hypnotherapy
16842 Von Karman Avenue, Suite 475
Irvine, CA 92714
1-714-261-6400

American Society of Clinical Hypnosis
2200 East Devon Avenue, Suite 291
Des Plaines, IL 60018
1-708-297-3317

Association for Applied Psychophysiology and
   Biofeedback
10200 West 44th Avenue, Suite 304
Wheat Ridge, CO 80033

Biofeedback Society of America
U.C.M.C. c268
4200 E. Ninth Avenue
Denver, CO 80262

Insight Meditation Society
1230 Pleasant Street
Barre, MA 01005
1-508-355-4378

Maharishi International University
1000 North Fourth Street
Fairfield, IA 52556
1-515-472-5031

NUTRITION

American Academy of Orthomolecular Medicine
900 North Federal Highway
Boca Raton, FL 33432
1-800-847-3802

American Association of Naturopathic Physicians
2366 Eastlake Avenue E, Suite 322
Seattle, WA 98102
1-206-323-7610

American Natural Hygiene Society
P.O. Box 30630
Tampa, FL 33630
1-813-855-6607

Institute for Natural Medicine
66½ North State Street
Concord, NH 03301
1-603-225-8844

NEWSLETTERS

Advanced Nutrition News with Dr. Ronald Hoffman
P.O. Box 1634
Rockville, ND 20850
1-888-267-7994
$29.95 per year. Published monthly. Call or write for a free three month trial subscripition.

Health Science Institute
105 West Monument Street
Baltimore, MD 21201
1-410-221-2600
$39.95 per year. Published monthly.

Health and Healing
7811 Montrose Road
Potomac, MD 20854
1-800-539-8219
$39.95 per year. Published monthly.

Second Opinion
1350 Center Drive
Dunwoody, GA 30328
1-770-668-0432
$39.95 per year. Published monthly.

❁

Appendix B:
Product Sources

Note: The MSM, ginger extracts, glucosamine, and chondroitan products are generally available at most health food stores, natural food stores, pharmacies, and occasionally, supermarkets, and are distributed by many different manufacturers. These items are also available over the Internet; simply type the appropriate keyword in the search box of your favorite search engines. None of the lists below represent an endorsement of any company, manufacturer, or distributor.

MSM

Most suppliers carry MSM in all its forms—capsules, powder, lotion, gel, spray, toothpaste—as well as products that contain MSM combined with vitamin C, bioflavonoids, and other nutrients.

Harvest Moon Natural Foods
2113A E. 151st Street
Olathe, KS 66062
1-888-437-2425
www.harvest-moon.com/msm/html

Natural Mom
www.naturalmom.com/MSMart.htm

SGS Research
14651 Oak Avenue
Irvine, CA 92606
714-651-6355
www.SuperGoodStuff.com

World Image Network
1-503-647-2244; or 503-647-0984 (fax)
e-mail: msm@worldimage.com

GINGER EXTRACT

Several companies specialize in ginger extract products. Zinaxin is available in the United States through one source only: FreeLife International, a multilevel marketing company. Under an exclusive agreement between the nutraceutical research company Eurovita International and FreeLife International, Zinaxin is sold exclusively by marketing executives of FreeLife International.

FreeLife International
333 Quarry Road
Milford, CT 06460
1-800-882-7240

New Chapter
www.newchapterinc.com/guide27.html

Pharmacy Express Ltd.
(For Zinaxin)
www.weblink.co.nz/FEX/FDpages/Zinax.html

Zinerin® forte
www.hankintatukku.com/Zinerin.html

GLUCOSAMINE AND CHONDROITAN

American Biologic
Chula Vista, CA

1-800-227-4458
(Produce chondroitin)

Great Earth
Ontario, CA
1-800-284-8243
(Produce glucosamine)

Jarrow Formulas
Los Angeles, CA
1-800-726-0886
(Produce glucosamine)

Nutramax
Baltimore, MD
1-800-925-5187
(Produce Cosamin DS, a combination of glucosamine and chondroitan)

TwinLab
Ronkonkoma, NY
1-800-645-5626
(Produce Joint Fuel, a combination of glucosamine and chondroitan; also, glucosamine and chondroitan separately)

Vitamin Research Products
Carson City, NV
1-800-877-2447
(Produce glucosamine and chondroitan)

Sources and Suggested Readings

Alman, Brian M. *Self-Hypnosis: The Complete Manual.* New York: Brunner/Mazel, 1992.

Arthritis Foundation. *Arthritis 101.* Marietta, GA: Longstreet Press, 1997.

Arthritis Today. September–October 1998.

Balch, James F., and Phyllis Balch. *Prescription for Nutritional Healing.* Garden City Park, NY: Avery Publishing Group, 1993.

Borysenko, Joan. *Minding the Body, Mending the Mind.* Toronto/New York: Bantam Books, 1988.

———. *The Power of the Mind to Heal.* Carson CA: Hay House, 1994.

Carper, Jean. *Food—Your Miracle Medicine.* New York: HarperCollins, 1993.

Christy, Martha M. *MSM: The Super Supplement*

of the Decade. Scottsdale: Wishland Publishing, 1997.

Duke, James A., Ph.D. *The Green Pharmacy*. New York: St. Martin's Press, 1997.

Epstein, Gerald. *Healing Visualizations*. New York: Bantam, 1989.

Eurovita. Company information on Zinaxin. Internet communication with Arne Skjold Iversen, M.D., November 1998.

Fezler, William. *Creative Imagery*. New York: Simon & Schuster, 1989.

Fisher, Stanley. *Discovering the Power of Self-Hypnosis*. New York: HarperCollins, 1991.

Fulder, Stephen. *The Ginger Book*. Garden City Park, NY: Avery Publishing, 1996.

Garrison, Robert, and Elizabeth Somer. *The Nutrition Desk Reference*. New Canaan, CT: Keats, 1995.

Goleman, Daniel, and Joel Gurin. *Mind Body Medicine: How to Use Your Mind for Better Health*. Yonkers, NY: Consumer Reports Books, 1993.

Green, Elmer. *Beyond Biofeedback*. New York: Delacorte, 1977.

Herschler, R.J. Personal correspondence. September 1998.

———. U.S. Patent 5,569,679; October 29, 1996.

———. U.S. Patent 4,512,421; 1985.

Hilgad, Ernest. *Hypnosis: In the Relief of Pain*. New York: Brunner/Mazel, 1994.

Jacob, S.W. "Preliminary Evaluation of MSM (dimethyl sulfone) in Osteoarthritis." Oregon Health Sciences University, 1 April 1997, unpublished paper.

Jacob, S.W., and R.J. Herschler. "Introductory Remarks: Dimethylsulfoxide After Twenty Years." *Ann NY Acad Sci* 1983; 411: xiii–xvii.

Kabat-Zinn, J. *Full Catastrophic Living: Using the Wisdom of Your Body and Mind to Face Stress, Pain, and Illness.* New York: Delacorte Press, 1990.

Lusk, Julie, ed. *30 Scripts for Relaxation, Imagery, and Inner Healing.* 2 vols. Duluth: Whole Person Associates, 1992.

McDonald, Kathleen. *How to Meditate.* Boston: Wisdom Publications, 1992.

Miller, Michael, M.D. *Therapeutic Hypnosis.* New York: Human Sciences Press, 1979.

Mindell, Earl L. *The MSM Miracle. Enhance Your Health With Organic Sulfur.* New Canaan, CT: Keats Publishing, 1997.

Moen, Larry, ed. *Guided Imagery.* 2 vols. Naples: United States Publishing, 1992.

Murray, M.T. *Arthritis: How You Can Benefit From Diet, Vitamins, Minerals, Herbs, Exercise, and Other Natural Methods.* Rocklin, CA: Prima Publishing, 1994.

Naparstek, Belleruth. *Staying Well with Guided Imagery.* New York: Time/Warner, 1994.

Pelletier, Kenneth R. *Mind as Healer, Mind as Slayer*. Rev. ed. New York: Delacorte, 1992.

Rossman, Martin L., M.D. *Healing Yourself: A Step-by-Step Program for Better Health Through Imagery*. New York: Walker & Co., 1987.

Samuels, Michael, M.D. *Healing With the Mind's Eye: A Guide for Using Imagery and Visions for Personal Growth and Healing*. New York: Simon & Schuster, 1990.

Sellnow, L. "MSM: An Aid from Nature." *The Blood Horse*, 6 June 1987.

Siegel, Bernie S., M.D. *Peace, Love & Healing: Bodymind Communication and the Path to Self-Healing*. New York: Harper & Row, 1989.

Siegel, J.M., and S.W. Jacob. "Current Status of MSM," 1996, unpublished paper. Oregon Health Sciences University, Portland, Oregon.

Srivastava, K., et al. "Ginger and Rheumatic Disorders." *Medical Hypothesis* 29:25–28, 1989.

Theodosakis, Jason. *The Arthritis Cure*. New York: St. Martin's, 1997.

Time/Life Books. *Drug and Natural Medicine Advisor*. Alexandria, VA: Editors of Time-Life Books, 1997.

Weil, Andrew, M.D. *Spontaneous Healing*. Boston: Houghton Mifflin, 1994.

Yates, John. *The Complete Book of Self-Hypnosis*. Chicago: Nelson- Hall, 1984.

Index

Deborah Mitchell is a medical writer and journalist specializing in natural medicine and nutrition topics. Her articles have appeared in professional journals as well as national consumer magazines. She has authored or co-authored nine books about various health topics, including *The Natural Health Guide to Headache Relief*, *The Dictionary of Natural Healing*, *Natural Aphrodisiacs*, and *The Broccoli Sprouts Breakthrough*. Ms. Mitchell lives and works in Tucson, Arizona.

Steven J. Bock, M.D., author of the foreword, is a traditionally trained physician who practices complementary medicine. In 1983 he and his brother, Kenneth Bock, M.D., founded the Rhinebeck (New York) Health Center for Progressive Medicine with the goal of providing the best of conventional medicine combined with the best of alternative therapies. He is the author of *Stay Young the Melatonin Way* and (with Kenneth Bock, M.D.) *Natural Relief for Your Child's Asthma*.

Alternative Healing Approaches

THE COMPLETE HERBAL COMPANION
Natural Solutions for You and Your Family
by Elizabeth Burch, N. D.
01385-4/$5.99 US/$7.99 Can

**MSM: THE NATURAL PAIN
RELIEF REMEDY**
by Deborah Mitchell
80899-4/$5.99 US/$7.99 Can

KAVA
NATURE'S STRESS RELIEF
by Kathryn M. Connor, M.D. and Donald S. Vaughan
80641-X/$5.99 US/$7.99 Can

ST. JOHN'S WORT
NATURE'S MOOD BOOSTER
*Everything You Need to Know about This
Natural Antidepressant*
by Michael E. Thase, M.D. and Elizabeth E. Loredo
80288-0/$5.99 US/$7.99 Can

GINKGO
NATURE'S BRAIN BOOSTER
by Alan H. Pressman, D.C., Ph.D., C.C.N.
with Helen Tracy
80640-1/$5.99 US/$7.99 Can

**A HANDBOOK OF NATURAL
FOLK REMEDIES**
by Elena Oumano, Ph.D.
78448-3/$5.99 US/$7.99 Can